# Welcome

Welcome to the most important journal of your life. Consider this the first step towards the future you have always dreamed of. Whether you are pursuing personal growth, rewarding relationships, career ambitions, greater prosperity, or any other aspirations, this book is your tool to making it all happen.

Manifestation helps you take control in a chaotic world by channelling your intentions towards your goals, but it's not simply about wishful thinking. The practice brings clarity and focus, turning your motivation into momentum so you can take action and make those dreams a reality.

In this journal, you'll learn all about this powerful practice and how to make it work for you, with plenty of practical advice on setting targets, overcoming obstacles and cultivating a growth mindset. Through a series of interactive exercises and prompts, you'll discover various techniques to support your manifestation, such as affirmations and visualisation. There is also a year's worth of diary entries to chart your progress. Here, you can take some time to reflect and realign each week, to help you stay on track.

Be open and honest with yourself, and be bold with your dreams. Your manifestation journey starts here…

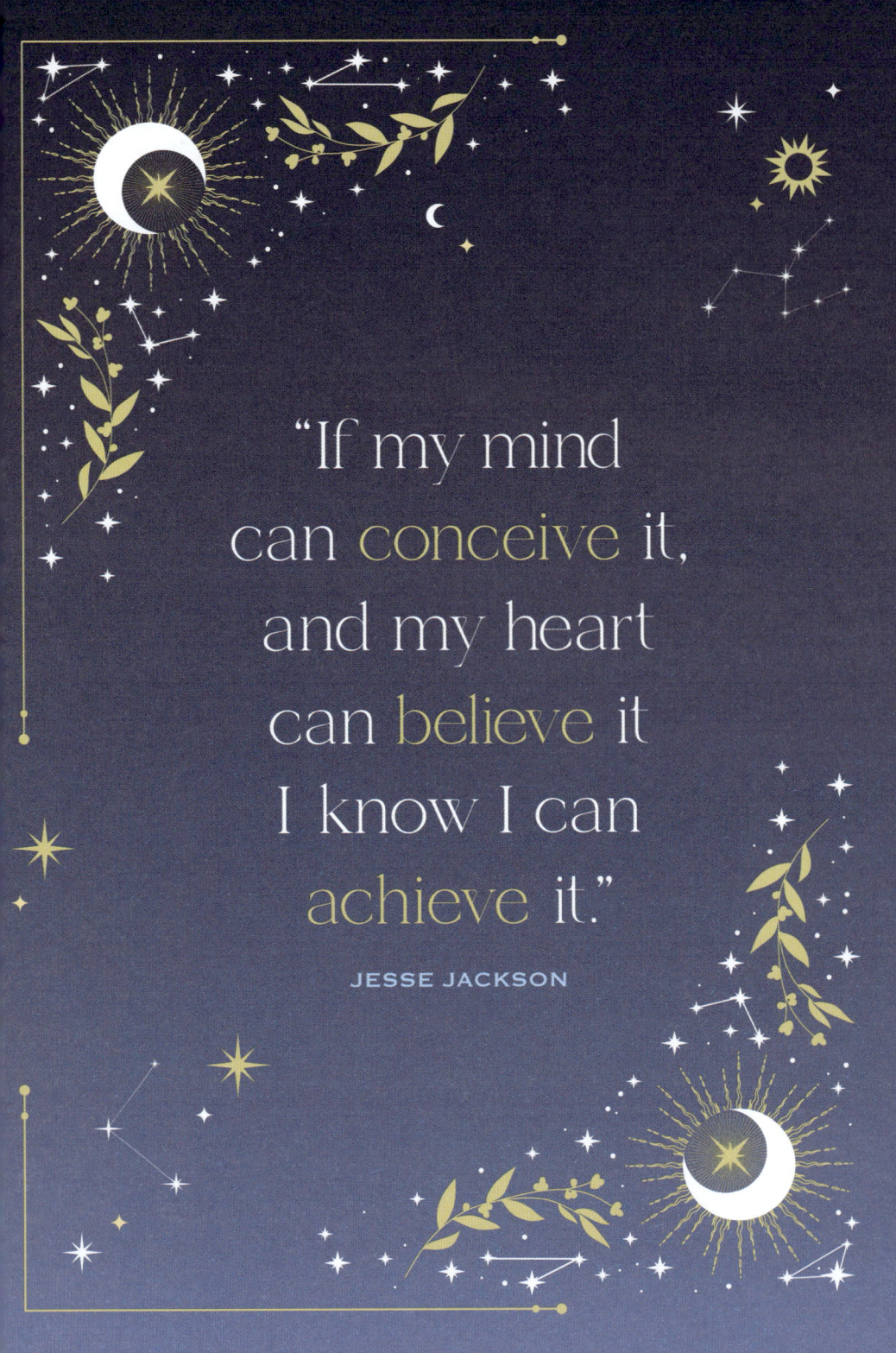

"If my mind can conceive it, and my heart can believe it I know I can achieve it."

JESSE JACKSON

# Contents

## 6
### UNDERSTANDING MANIFESTATION
Learn more about this practice and discover how to make it work for you

## 48
### INTERACTIVE EXERCISES
A series of prompts and activities to encourage awareness and reflection

## 76
### YOUR JOURNAL
Chart your manifestation experiences and progress in this 52-week diary

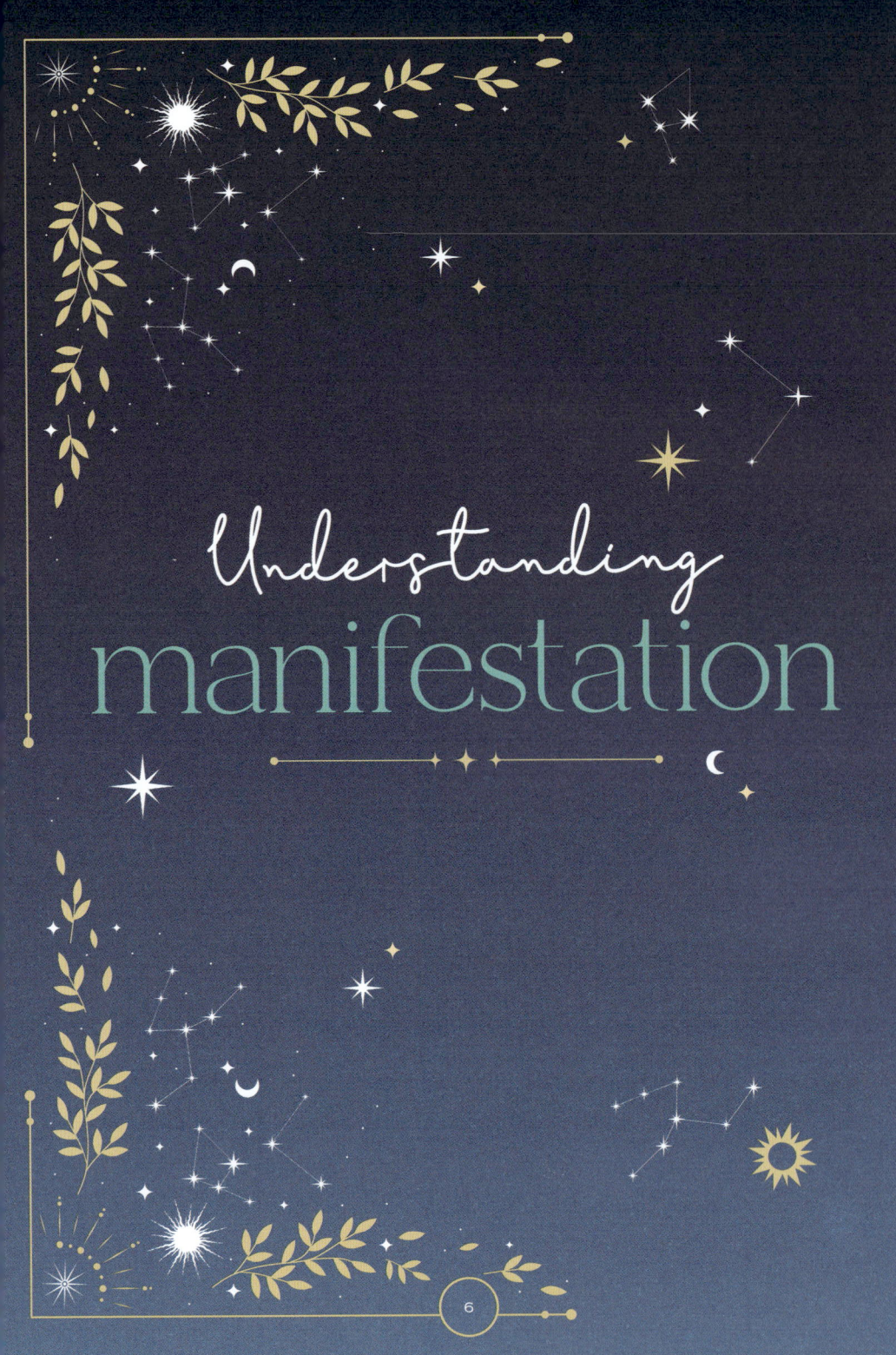

# Understanding manifestation

| | |
|---|---|
| 8 | WHAT IS MANIFESTATION? |
| 14 | THE SCIENCE OF MANIFESTATION |
| 20 | TYPES OF MANIFESTING |
| 28 | TURN INTENTION INTO ACTION |
| 32 | OVERCOMING OBSTACLES |
| 38 | YOUR MANIFESTATION GOALS |
| 44 | COMPLEMENTARY PRACTICES |

# What is manifestation?

**HOW MODERN MANIFESTATION GREW FROM ANCIENT ORIGINS INTO THE PRINCIPLES WE CAN FOLLOW TODAY**

WORDS | JULIE BASSETT

Can the power of positive thought change your life for the better? That's the principle behind manifestation, a belief that you can be successful and meet your goals by focusing your thoughts and actions on turning your hopes and dreams into reality.

This is not a new concept, though it has gained fresh popularity in recent times. In fact, the roots of manifestation can be traced back to the ancient world. The idea that our thoughts can influence our lived reality has been woven throughout spiritual, cultural and religious beliefs for centuries. Manifestation is linked to 'magical thinking', which is a belief that our own thoughts and actions can influence events in the world; within religion, prayer is often used to ask a deity to influence events in the world, while manifestation comes from within ourselves.

Hermeticism, which is based on ancient texts known collectively as the *Hermetica*, covers a wide range of philosophical concepts, religious traditions and esoteric teachings that date back to ancient Egypt and Greece. The *Hermetica* was attributed to the legendary figure Hermes Trismegistus, and had a huge influence on the cultures of these ancient civilisations. Many of the key principles of Hermeticism are deeply rooted in manifestation. These ideas were passed down through spiritual teachings for many hundreds of years, and later compiled into a book called *The Kybalion* in 1908, which has formed the basis of many New Thought and New Age principles. In *The Kybalion*, the Hermetic philosophy is condensed into seven universal principles, the first of which is 'The principle of mentalism', which teaches that the mind is a powerful creative force, shaping the reality that we experience around us. Another key element is 'The principle of vibration', which forms a core concept in the law of attraction, which we'll explore in a moment.

Hinduism also has spiritual beliefs similar to modern-day manifestation. Karma follows the law of cause and effect (which is also one of the principles of Hermeticism outlined in *The Kybalion*). That is, your actions, emotions and thoughts have consequences that influence your life's outcome. Good actions

## The roots of manifestation can be traced back to the ancient world

give you positive karma, and building up good karma determines your future destiny; only you are responsible for your choices and hence the consequences. In Buddhism, the focus is on intention and action. In order to manifest the life you want, you need to take steps towards that outcome, led by positive intentions and thoughts. All of these ideas feed into what we understand of manifestation today.

Manifestation took another leap forward through the New Thought religious movement in the early 19th century, which brought together the teachings from many ancient religions and philosophies, including the ones we've mentioned here. One of the core beliefs of New Thought is that thoughts, beliefs and actions can directly impact our reality, and the mind has influence over the body. It focuses on the power of positive thinking to shape our own experiences and our experience of the world.

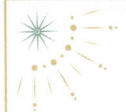

The law of attraction came out of this period of New Thought in the later 19th century, with a number of important books and essays presenting the concept to the world. This philosophy is based on the idea that our positive thoughts attract positive experiences, while negative thoughts attract negative experiences. Therefore, if we want to meet our goals and desires, we need to focus positively on the outcome we want and we will be successful. The law of attraction can be applied to any aspect of our lives, from happiness and health to relationships and finances. The core idea is that 'like attracts like', so when you give out optimism, joy and passion, you attract other people who are on the same 'wavelength' who bring that same energy back to you.

In the 20th century, the law of attraction gained traction and there was a lot of interest in these ideas. *Think and Grow Rich*, published in 1937, remains a bestseller. Its principles of success, in particular financial success, being based around a positive mindset and focused thought were derived from the law of attraction. In 2006, the film *The Secret* brought the New Thought ideas and the law of attraction to a new audience. The documentary was made up of interviews that vouched for the law of attraction in action across all aspects of life. The film was turned into a book that went on to sell more than 30 million copies, introducing even more people to the power of manifestation.

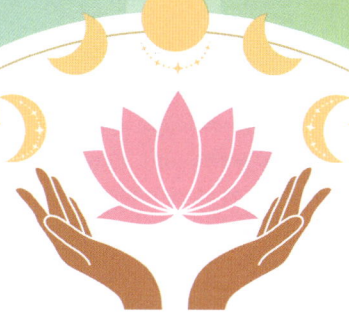

# The role of mindset

Manifestation only works if you have the right mindset, and whether you have a fixed or growth mindset. A fixed mindset is when you believe that your personal traits and abilities are incapable of significant change or development. Someone with a fixed mindset is more likely to avoid challenges, because they don't believe they can overcome them and are afraid of failure. They may stick within their comfort zone and never believe that they can move beyond it. Someone with a growth mindset, however, believes they can develop throughout their life. This person will thrive on challenges as an opportunity to learn, and will see failure as a setback from which they can grow.

Manifestation requires strong belief, and you need to be open minded and willing to embrace the possibilities. In order for manifestation to be a success for you, you need to be willing to shift your mindset and address your limiting beliefs. It means embracing an abundance mindset, which means believing that there are enough possibilities for everyone – rather than thinking that someone else's success limits your own ability to achieve the same (as in a scarcity mindset). This might feel a bit uncomfortable or scary at first, especially if you have a negative or fixed mindset, but the more you practise the art of manifestation, the more you can shift your mindset towards prosperity.

## Modern-day manifestation

And so, we come to today where manifestation has developed into a practice that can enhance our health and wellbeing. The interest in manifestation has been growing rapidly since the Covid-19 pandemic in 2020, seemingly fuelled by a desire to find control and meaning in our lives amid the backdrop of a chaotic environment. Internet searches for 'manifesting' went up 600% in early 2020, introducing an eager new audience to the principles of the theory, still rooted in those deep ancient origins.

The concept is simple: think positively and with intention, and your hopes, goals and dreams can become reality through meaningful action. Think negatively, and you're limiting your possibilities and preventing your goals and dreams from manifesting. There are limitations, of course. We exist within the laws of the universe and natural order – you can't manifest a physical object into being, but you could manifest a happier and stronger relationship or the next step in your career path. Not only that, we exist within the limitations of our own minds and what we believe we're capable of, which is why having the right mindset and being open to possibility is important when it comes to the success of manifestation.

> Manifestation can be an effective tool for personal development and growth

This might all sound a bit too magical or too good to be true, but while the roots of the practice may be deeply spiritual, once you get to grips with the practical applications, you'll see that the idea of manifestation is closely linked with success in many ways. Think of those top-end athletes who talk about visualising themselves crossing the finish line first as a way of manifesting a win. Or the business entrepreneur who knows exactly how they see the next year, five years and ten years unfolding into a successful venture. Manifestation isn't just about belief – if you simply believe that you will find your dream job, then it might not happen. But if you channel that belief into action, making choices and decisions that are driven by what you want to achieve, then you can bring your goal into reality.

Manifestation can be an effective tool for personal development and growth. Rather than being stuck in a cycle of negative thinking, perfectionism, low self-esteem and anxiety, manifestation techniques teach you how to focus on your values, to align your lifestyle with your beliefs, and to channel positive thought into your actions. It also enables you to reframe negative experiences, helping you to process and cope with them, diverting that energy back into action and intention. Regular manifestation can nurture self-confidence, optimism, hope and joy. It can also help with our mental wellbeing, replacing negative self-talk with acceptance and self-love.

As with any wellness trend, the art of manifestation has grown, and you can now attend courses, retreats and seminars to unlock its secrets. However, it doesn't have to be that complicated, as we'll teach you step by step throughout this journal, including the science behind why manifestation works and how to incorporate it into your life. We'll provide interactive exercises to help bring clarity and focus to your intentions and goals. Manifestation sits comfortably alongside other wellness practices, like journalling, meditation, mindfulness and showing gratitude, which we'll also explore in more detail in this journal. Manifestation is a personal practice and, once you learn the basics, it's something you can incorporate into your daily life simply and effectively.

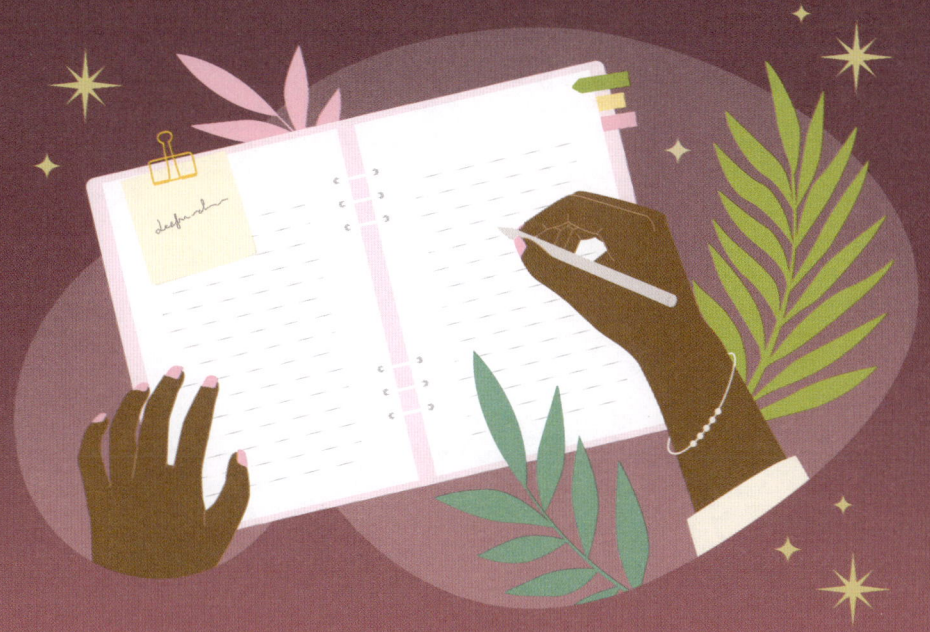

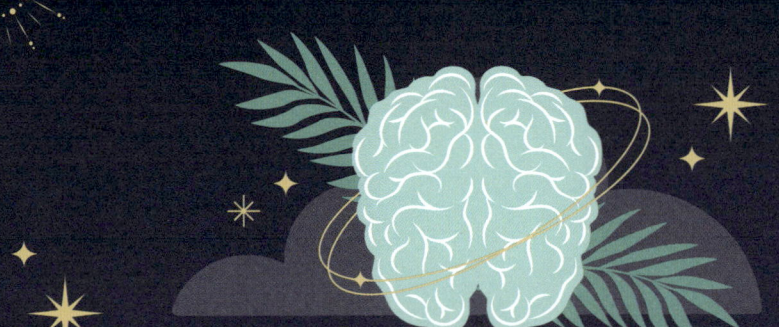

# The science of manifestation

**WE DELVE INTO THE PSYCHOLOGY AND NEUROSCIENCE THAT EXPLAINS WHY MANIFESTATION WORKS**

WORDS | JULIE BASSETT

It's easy to dismiss the idea of manifestation as magical, or even wishful, thinking. Social media doesn't help its cause sometimes, with accounts suggesting that you simply have to believe that a massive cheque will land in your lap, and lo and behold, there it is. It relegates manifestation to seemingly pseudoscience and irrational thinking. However, true manifestation – that is, a combination of both intention and action – is backed by science.

To truly understand how manifestation works, you need to separate the fact from the fantastical. There are many misconceptions of what manifestation is, the most common being that you can manifest anything you want simply because you will it to be so. This makes manifestation a passive activity; you don't have to do anything, you just have to think it. Of course, it would be great if that were the case, but sadly this idea stretches the bounds of reality.

Another misconception is that there are rules to how you manifest – a belief that if you don't do your daily affirmations, for example, it will never happen.

There is no one way to manifest; you will learn a set of tools that can help you to unlock the power of your own brain, but which tools work will vary from person to person.

If you want to introduce manifestation into your life, then you're not going to find the right way forward through anecdotes, pseudoscience and magical beliefs. Instead, look towards the world of science to understand how the brain works, and see how we can leverage that to make our dreams a reality.

## What does the science say?

By learning about both psychology (the scientific study of mind and behaviour) and neuroscience (the scientific study of the nervous system), we can learn more about why and how manifestation can – and does – work.

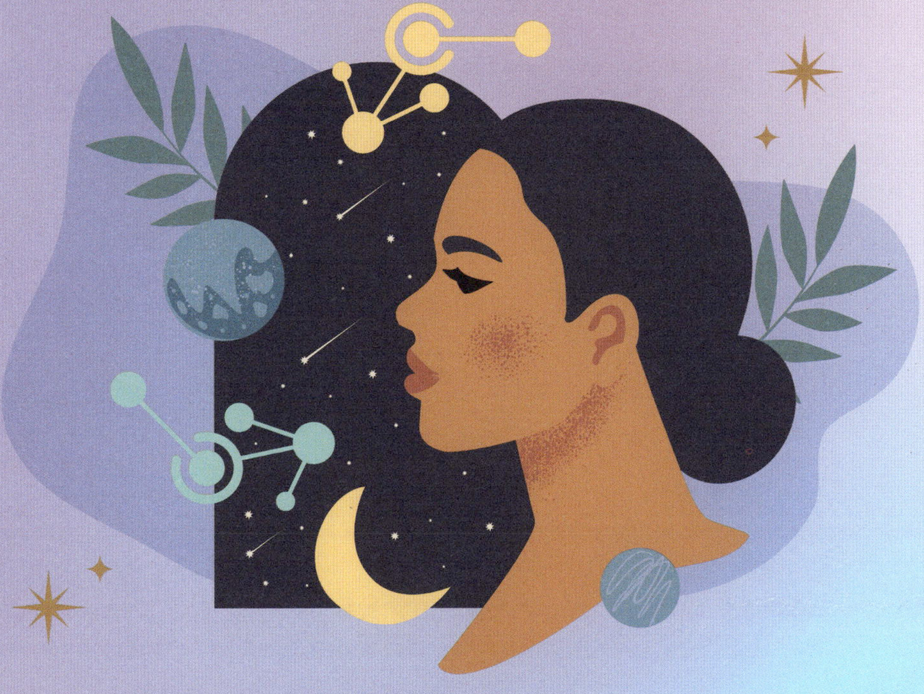

The reticular activating system (RAS) is a network of nerves located in the brainstem. It regulates our wakefulness, alertness and attention. It helps us to sift through the sheer volume of information we receive every day, processing

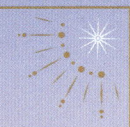

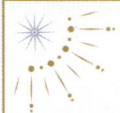

it to enable the important data to get through. It determines what is important based on what we're focused on, our internal belief system, and our goals.

This is linked into the idea of 'selective attention', with RAS acting as the filter for information. Selective attention is a skill we all use every day, without really realising. For example, when you're having a conversation with someone in a noisy environment, your brain will naturally attempt to filter out the background chatter to help you hone in on what they are saying.

Selective attention can help explain a little about why manifestation works. You know that feeling when something specific is on your mind, such as how much you'd love to learn a new skill, then suddenly you see adverts for that skill everywhere you go, or a friend mentions it in conversation, or it crops up on television? We often put this down to sheer coincidence – how strange that we're now seeing the very thing we're thinking about all the time! But selective attention means that when you focus on something you want to achieve, your brain will start actively seeking out ways to deliver that outcome and filter out distractions. What you're seeing around you would always have been there, but caught up among lots of other stimuli; when you focus your attention on a

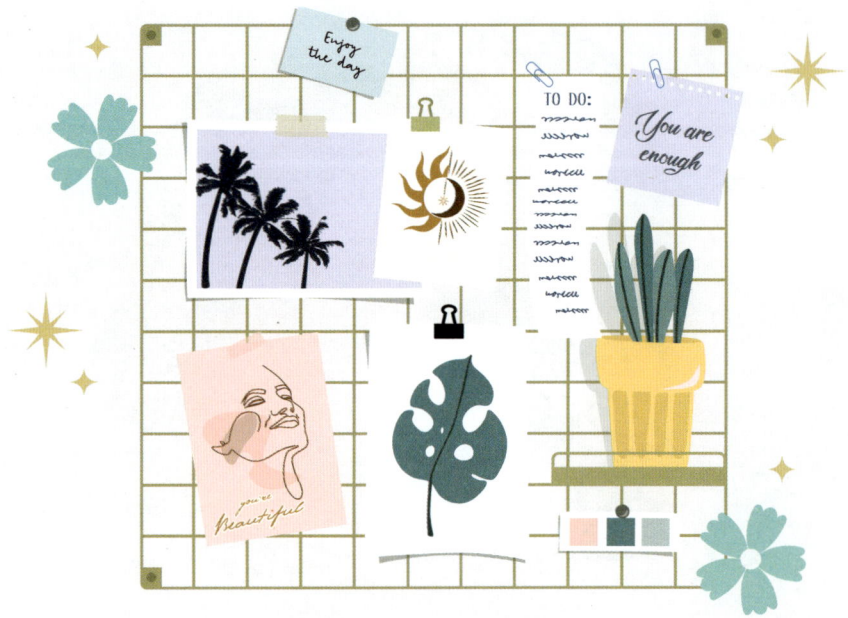

goal, you start to zone in on all the relevant information in your environment. If one of your goals is to find a new job, for example, once you've established your goal and set your mind on it, your attention will become more focused on seeking out opportunities to help you make that next step.

Manifestation, therefore, can be used to help train your RAS and use your inherent selective attention skills to focus on your specific goals and desires. By setting your intentions, your brain will seek out relevant opportunities and

> Selective attention is a skill we all use every day, without really realising

information based on this new point of focus, which makes it more likely that you will achieve the outcome you want. Training your RAS takes time and effort, through repeated focus on your goals. This is why manifestation practices, like visualisation techniques, mood boards and regular positive affirmations, can help – they keep you focused and help your RAS to learn what's important.

This idea of taking control of your attention and where it's directed is not a new concept. Back in 1890, William James wrote in *The Principles of Psychology* that attention is "taking possession by the mind, in clear and vivid form, of one out of what seem several simultaneously possible objects of thought… It implies withdrawal from some things in order to deal effectively with others". You can prime your brain each day by repeating your goals or affirmations, so that it's ready to pay attention on the right areas of focus.

## The power of the mind

There is a strong link between our thoughts and beliefs, and how they can manifest and impact on the real world. You have probably heard of the placebo effect, which is when a person's physical or mental health improves even when receiving a fake (placebo) treatment because of a strong belief in the outcome of the treatment. This belief creates a connection between the mind and body, and in some cases can even trigger the brain to help combat symptoms that are under its control, such as the perception of pain or stress.

## Positive thinking can lead to better performance and better outcomes

This concept links into the power of our thoughts and how they manifest into reality. Everything we do starts with a thought. If you think about making a cup of tea, you'll be able to put that into action and do it. This goes deeper too. If you think in a positive way, you're inviting positivity into your life. We know that having a positive mental attitude (PMA), or a positive mindset, can help you reach your goals. Positive thinking can lead to better performance and better outcomes.

One way to tap into this is through visualisation – creating imagery in the mind around a desired outcome. One study* explains that: "Imagery is a mental performance improvement technique that involves 'programming' body and mind with the purpose of responding optimally in a performance situation." The use of visualisation has been shown to be effective in academic, athletic, and work contexts. Positive thinking can also impact those around us, as well as enhancing our own self-belief. The Pygmalion effect is a known psychological phenomenon where having high expectations can lead to improved performance in others. When we have high expectations of others, we act in a way that encourages or supports that person. This impacts their self-belief, which then helps them to take positive actions, which reflect back on us and influence our own self-belief, and our actions towards others.

The reason this all works is that we're able to tap into our brain and make changes to its structure. Our brains are in a constant state of development; it is reshaped and adapted as we go through life in response to what we experience and learn. This is called neuroplasticity, where the brain can 'reorganise', strengthening neural connections. Take, for example, when we want to learn a new language or play a musical instrument. We practise over and over again, and as we do, the brain is working on strengthening our neural pathways and building new connections until we can master the skill. Neuroplasticity is crucial to manifestation – when you set your intentions and focus on them repeatedly, your brain will build those neural connections to help you achieve your goals. Being

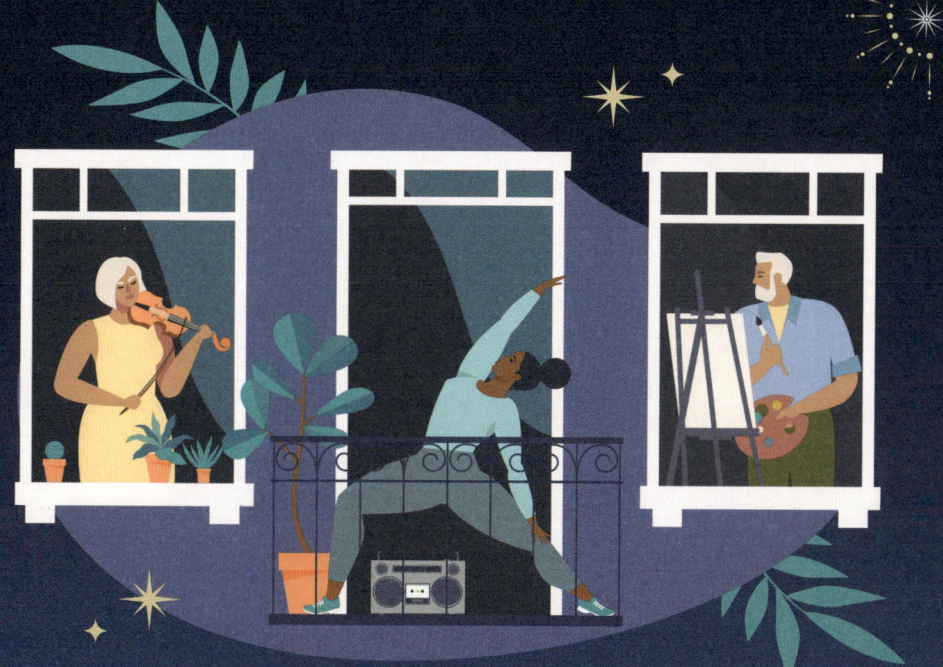

intentional about your thoughts and your attention makes your brain realise that this is something that's important and should be prioritised. In turn, this can boost your motivation and positivity, so you seek out opportunities and feel driven to strive for what you want.

There are limitations, however. You can't discount the impact that external influences have on the outcome of your intentions. Dr James R Doty, a Stanford neurosurgeon and neuroscientist, is one of the foremost experts on the science of manifestation, and he explains that manifestation is about maximising our ability to turn dreams into reality, but understanding that there are no guarantees. In a 2024 podcast, he said: "What we're talking about [is] 'what are the mechanisms and the actions I have to take to maximise my ability to manifest?' But there are other external circumstances that impact, and it may be that you are not aware of certain things that are impeding your progress, or there are other larger things that are having an effect."

Over the next few pages, we'll be diving deep into the tools you can utilise to maximise your ability to manifest, as well as how to turn intention into action. By practising these, and finding the tools that are best suited to you, you can make neural changes in the brain that will keep you motivated and focused on meeting your goals.

*Blankert T, Hamstra MR. Imagining Success: Multiple Achievement Goals and the Effectiveness of Imagery. *Basic Appl Soc Psych*, 2017 Jan 2.

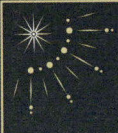

# Types of manifesting

**MANIFESTATION IS ABOUT HAVING A CLEAR FOCUS AND THE RIGHT TOOLS TO SET YOUR INTENTIONS**

WORDS | JULIE BASSETT

While you can choose to apply manifestation to any goal or desire, for most people, they tend to fall into one of a few key areas.

## Health and wellbeing

Wellness is a common area of focus, whether that's in terms of your physical or mental wellbeing. For example, you may be very busy and under a lot of stress, and feel that as a result you're not living your life in a way that's authentic to your true self. Maybe this has led to you feeling unwell, or not prioritising self-care or movement, and it's impacting on your sleep. You may wish to manifest a calmer lifestyle where you are in control of your time and able to set clear boundaries, as well as feel more at peace and able to nourish your body with what it needs to feel good. You could use visualisation techniques to create an image of the person you want to be, which can help you set clear intentions. What does that person feel like, what do they do to achieve that feeling, what is different in their life compared to your life now? This helps you to set more specific goals that bring you closer to the person you want to become, and enables you to align your actions to meet those goals.

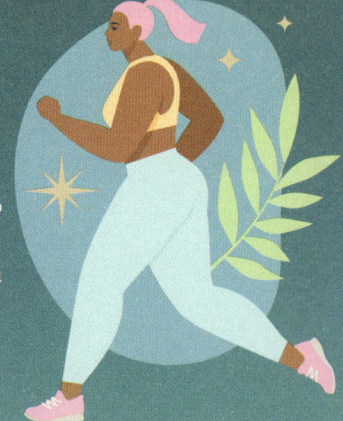

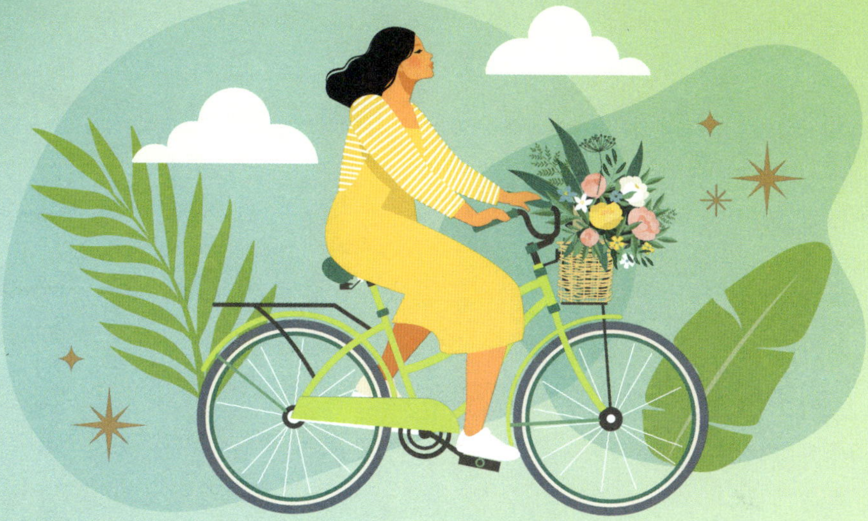

> Believe that what you're looking for is out there and that you don't have to settle for anything less

## Happiness and fulfilment

You may want to focus more on your own happiness and experience a sense of fulfilment, where you feel you have purpose. This can mean thinking about what's important to you in terms of your beliefs, your world view, your politics, your social connections, your relationships – learning who you are or who you want to be. Sometimes there isn't a specific and tangible end goal, but more an ongoing desire to feel content and at peace, knowing that you're living in alignment with your values. A good way to manifest this can be through the use of affirmations, which are tailored to your personal values and how you want to interact with the world. With these affirmations in mind, they can influence the decisions and interactions you make throughout the day. For example, if happiness to you means being kind to others, you might affirm this by helping someone in trouble or doing a random act of kindness, which then manifests the happiness you seek.

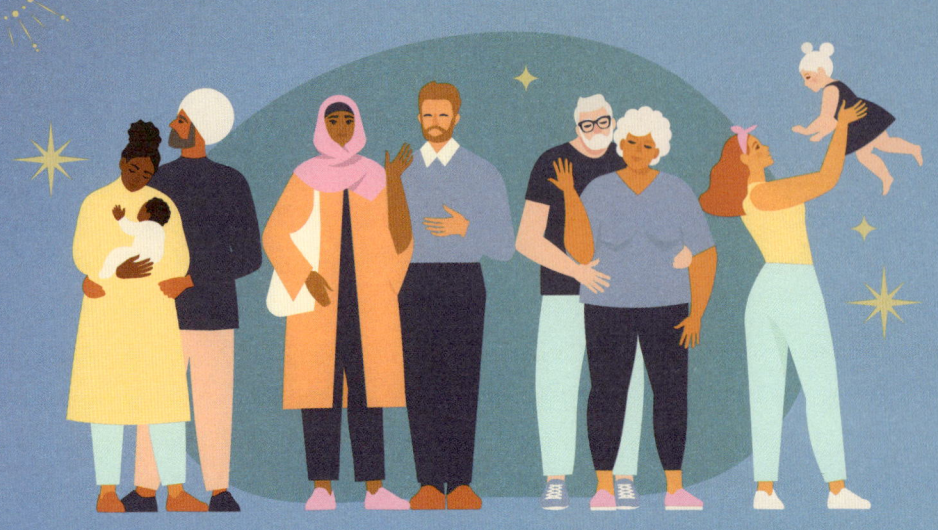

*Affirmations are reminders of who you are and what you can achieve*

## Relationships

Many people turn to manifestation for their relationships, whether that's in terms of building a trusted friendship or having an enriching romantic partnership. It starts with being very specific about your intentions and having a clear idea of what you want from a relationship. How do you want to feel (loved, safe, trusted), what qualities would your partner have (kindness, generosity, humour), and what would the relationship be like (equal, passionate, comfortable)? Once you have this tangible outline, you can align your emotions to be open for this relationship to come along and to know that you're worthy of it. When you meet someone, trust your inner instincts – does this person have the qualities you're looking for to get the outcome you desire? You need to believe that what you're looking for is out there and that you don't have to settle for anything less. This will make you more purposeful in your decisions – if something isn't working in a relationship, have the courage to walk away. When you're truly aligned with your desires and focused on what you're looking for, you're more likely to attract the right person into your life.

## Wealth and abundance

Another very common focus area for manifestation is for good fortune, in particular around money, though it could be other forms of wealth. Sadly, it's not enough to just hope for more money; you need to be very clear about your intentions and goals in order to manifest a situation that will help you reach your financial goals. What level of wealth do you want to achieve that would enable you to live your life in the way you want to? What is enough to be comfortable and reduce worry or pressure? Once you have this number in your head, you can align your thoughts and visualise the life you want to have. Having this clear in your mind will drive you to take action – you might be motivated to apply for a promotion or a new job with a higher salary, when you would previously have held back; or you might approach your spending with a more mindful attitude, deciding whether each purchase is in line with your future financial goals.

## Take action

With any form of manifestation, it takes both intention and action, as well as being specific and clear with what you desire. You can tap into different techniques to help with this. Some techniques might work better within different focus areas, and you may just feel more drawn to some than others. We outline some of the main techniques used in manifestation in the following pages, but however you choose to manifest, the key is to make sure you build it into your life routinely so that it becomes a habit. Regular practice also helps to cultivate a mindset that leaves you open to opportunity and success.

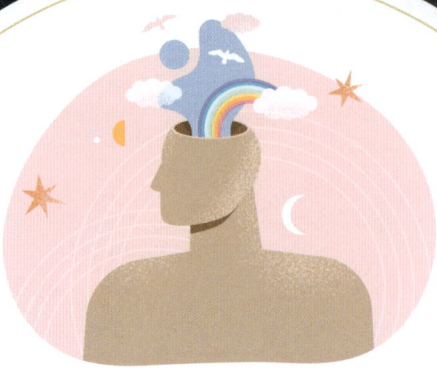

# Visualisation

**WHAT IS IT?**

This is a technique that involves using your imagination to picture your desired outcome or goal in detail, and then helps you to set your intentions.

**HOW TO DO IT:**

Many of us know what we want to manifest, but we can't always see what that looks like. Tapping into the power of visualisation helps you to focus on the details and gain clarity on what you're seeking. As well as visualising the outcome, you can imagine yourself going through the different steps that you need to take to reach your goal. Because your mind has already seen the outcome, it will then be primed ready to seek out opportunities that align with the mental image. It's a creative process, which can help your brain to be ready to find inventive solutions to help you manifest your goals. It also helps with self-esteem and confidence, because you've already 'seen' what it takes to accomplish what you want.

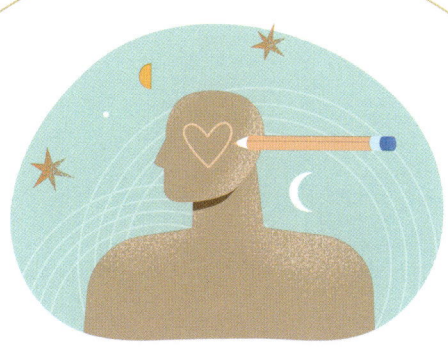

# Scripting

**WHAT IS IT?**

Scripting is a technique where you write down your goals or desires in the present tense, as if they've already been achieved.

**HOW TO DO IT:**

Some people work better with visuals, but others are better with words. If you're someone who finds it difficult to build mental pictures, give this method a go instead. It's similar to journalling, but where that is about reflecting on your day based on present reality, scripting encourages you to put yourself in the place of your future self. When we usually write down our goals, we write in the future tense, such as "I hope that in the future I will be in a strong and loving relationship"; in scripting, however, you are already in that relationship and you would write about how that feels in the present tense. It can seem a bit 'out there' at first, but it helps you to focus on what you're looking for and why you're looking for it, which will consequently motivate you to take opportunities towards that point.

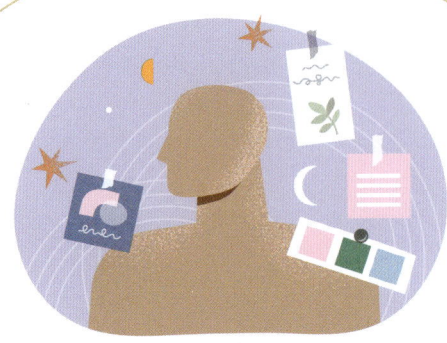

# Mood boards

**WHAT IS IT?**

Otherwise known as vision boards, mood boards are another type of visualisation technique, but one that's more tangible.

**HOW TO DO IT:**

Mood boards are collages that are made up of photos, words, imagery, quotes and more that reflect your true desires and values. They are designed to be an inspiration and motivation for what you're working towards. The act of putting a mood board together is a mindful one and can help you develop a clearer vision of what you want to achieve. First you need to gather material for it, which you can do online or via magazines, leaflets and brochures. Pick what you're drawn to and what you feel truly reflects what you want in your future. You then use the material to create a poster or digital collage with all of these things on (print a copy out if it's online). This should then be placed somewhere where you'll see it regularly so it's always fresh in your mind to keep you open to opportunity.

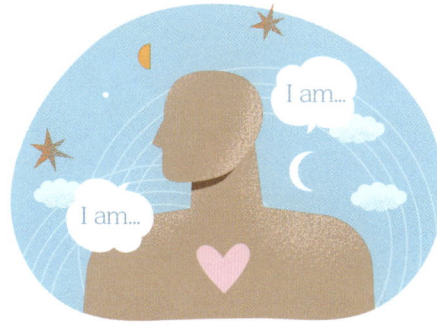

# Affirmations

**WHAT IS IT?**

Affirmations are short, positive statements that help to align your mindset and empower you to manifest your goals.

**HOW TO DO IT:**

You might already be familiar with what is meant by affirmations. These statements are essentially reminders of who you are and what you are capable of achieving. Like scripting, they should be set in the present tense and repeated daily to help encourage a more positive and opportunistic growth mindset. Your affirmations should be specific to your goals in order to be truly effective, and they should focus on what you want or desire, and not what you don't want. For example, rather than saying "I'm going to try to avoid unhealthy food today", you could instead say "I honour my body by nourishing it with healthy food" – by repeating this positive statement, your mind will believe it to already be true, and you will therefore make positive decisions that align with the affirmation.

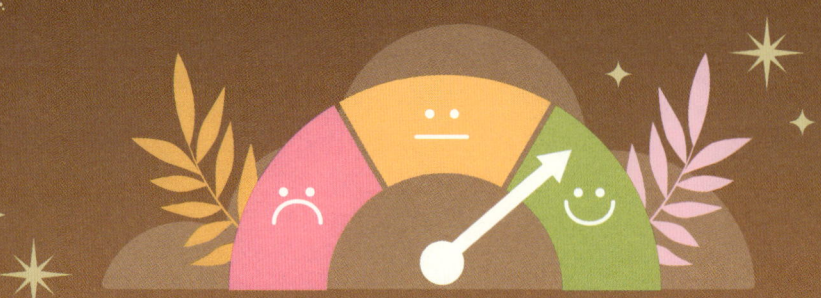

# Turn intention *into* action

### HOW TO TAKE POSITIVE AND PROACTIVE STEPS TOWARDS MANIFESTING YOUR GOALS
#### WORDS | JULIE BASSETT

The first step to manifesting is thinking about what you intend to achieve. Hopefully, by this stage, you will have come up with an idea of what you desire, and maybe even thought about which manifestation methods you feel most drawn to. That said, it can be hard to know what to do next, because the gap between where you are right now and where you want to be can feel insurmountable.

It's a good idea to put your intentions down on paper. By taking the time to address your goals in writing, it helps you to streamline your focus. We have some advice on how to create effective goals and intentions later in this journal (starting on page 38). It can be useful to have your goals written down in a small notebook that you can carry around with you, such as this journal, to act as a tangible reminder every day of what you're working towards.

Your end goal can feel a long way off, which doesn't help with staying motivated and on track. It's better to break your goal down into smaller, more manageable steps and specific actions that you need to take to stay on the path towards the end result. For example, if you're looking to manifest your dream job, one of your mini goals might be to undergo some extra training or earn qualifications that enable you to prepare for the role. You might then break that down further into action points, such as researching available training courses, identifying the right course, applying for the course, putting the course dates in your diary, blocking out time for any revision or prep you need to do, and so on. Some people like to have these actions listed out in a checkbox format, so you can tick each task off as you complete it. This can help a great deal with motivation and keep you moving forward.

The other important factor is ensuring you're in the right mindset. Your mind is a powerful tool and it's what can help turn your intentions into actions. The well-known saying, "The body achieves what the mind believes" is very apt; our thoughts and beliefs can directly influence the actions we physically take. You need to believe in yourself and that you're capable of turning your dreams into reality. This is where the manifestation techniques come into play. Things like visualisation and affirmations help to maintain a positive and

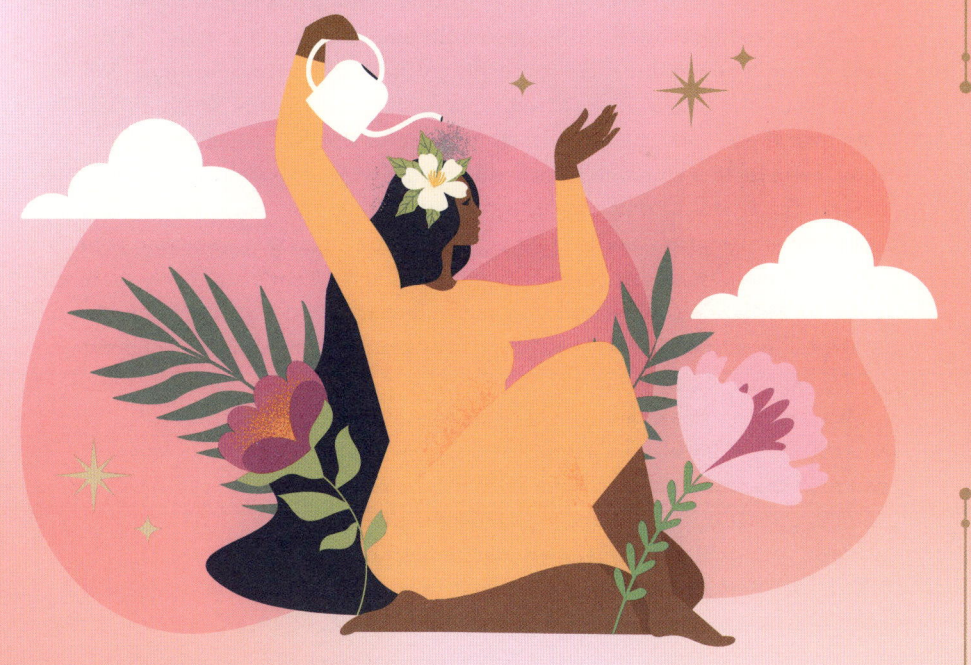

## "The body achieves what the mind believes"

goal-driven mindset. It can be hard to always maintain a positive mindset, especially when you feel as though it's taking too long to meet the goals you've set. Sometimes it feels like you're making no progress, but if you have made your plan of action, and you're ticking things off step by step, then you are moving in the right direction.

The best way to maintain a positive mindset is to ensure you do your manifestation practices regularly and often – ideally every day. You're looking to create a habit, and in order for something to become a habit you need to be consistent. Try to do your manifestation practises at the same time every day, at a time that suits you best. For example, many people like to do affirmations first thing in the morning to set them up for the day. You may want to have your manifestations written out somewhere where you will see them, such as stuck to a mirror you use in the mornings, and set aside five minutes every day to run through them. One top tip for creating a new habit is to attach it to something you already do without even thinking about it. For example, you probably don't even think about brushing your teeth in the mornings – you just do it! You could attach your affirmations to the mirror in the bathroom and read over them, committing yourself to them for the day, as you're cleaning your teeth. By stacking one habit onto another, you're less likely to forget and, before long, it will be part of your everyday routine.

Once manifestation has become a daily practice, this will help train your mind to remain in a positive and proactive mindset. That's not to say there will never be setbacks; some days are going to be harder than others, but by having an overall positive mindset, you'll find it easier to get back on track knowing you're capable of achieving your goal.

Manifestation is a combination of both intention and action, but it's also an act of self-belief. When you're in the right mindset, your mind will be more open to opportunity, enabling you to take active steps towards your goal. But remember, manifestation doesn't happen overnight; it takes consistent, repeated action, perseverance and patience.

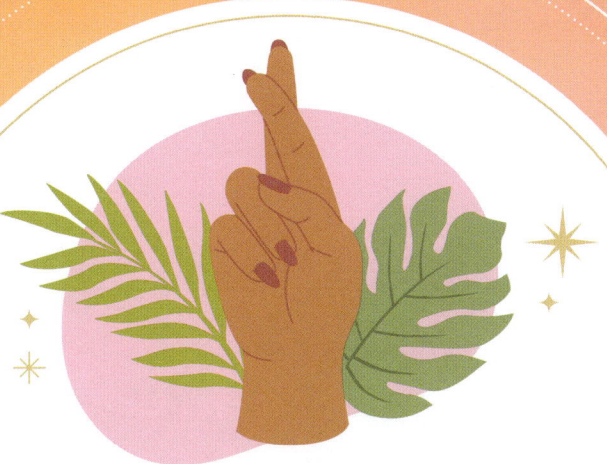

# Common pitfalls

If you're new to manifestation, beware of common missteps that can hold you back and make it harder to turn your goals into reality. One of the most common is confusing manifestation with wishful thinking. Wishful thinking is when you believe something to be true, or will come true, simply because you wish it so. It isn't based upon evidence or facts, and disregards the effort you need to put in to true manifestation. You may wish to feel in good health, but unless you take action to change bad habits or address the underlying causes of poor health, nothing will ultimately change. If you rely on wishful thinking, opportunities might pass you by as you're not primed to be watching out for them. Waiting for good things to come your way just leads to disappointment. Rather, you need to actively create an environment that attracts good things to you, so you're ready to embrace them. Another common problem is letting negative thoughts, or a lack of self-belief, hold you back and undo your hard work. Learning to challenge and overcome these thoughts is a skill, as we'll explain in the next section.

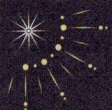
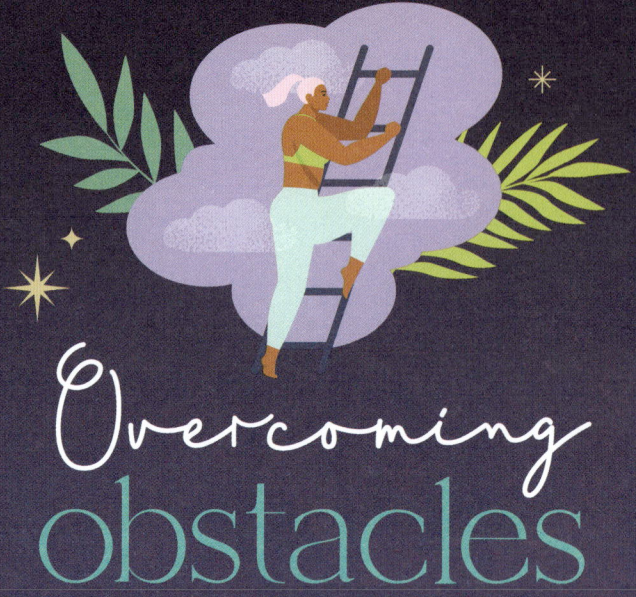

# Overcoming obstacles

**LEARN HOW TO IDENTIFY YOUR BLOCKS AND MOVE THROUGH THEM TO MANIFEST YOUR DREAMS**

WORDS | JOSE HALL

As with any practice, sometimes we encounter obstacles that feel difficult to overcome. This is a natural part of your manifestation journey that can be worked *with* to aid you in moving forwards and achieving your goals. By cultivating awareness and learning how to shift our mindset, we can turn these blocks into opportunities for growth. As sporting legend Michael Jordan once said, "Obstacles don't have to stop you. If you run into a wall, don't turn around and give up. Figure out how to climb it, go through it, or work around it."

## Identifying your obstacles

Before you can overcome your blocks, you first need to recognise them. By identifying these obstacles and understanding where they come from, you can begin the process of shifting your mindset and aligning with your desires.

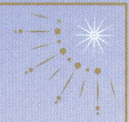

Perhaps the most common obstacle is having a loud 'inner critic' that engages in negative self-talk and reinforces limiting beliefs. This might present in recurring thoughts such as "I'm not good enough" or "It won't work for me", and if left unchallenged it can foster a general state of scepticism and a lack of belief in yourself and the practice of manifestation.

Another obstacle that can really get in the way of manifesting our desires is fear, particularly a fear of failure. If you are constantly worrying about not succeeding in your goals then you may start to feel a sense of pre-emptive disappointment, which can lead to resistance, and a tendency to stay within your comfort zone. Attachment to outcomes can also become a barrier to our practice. However much we might wish we could, we can't control *how* or *when* things manifest – and trying to can negatively impact results. This, along with many of the obstacles that arise in your manifestation practice, can often be linked back to a subconscious conditioning – ideas that we picked up in childhood, or approaches we've developed as ways of coping with difficult experiences.

Complementary practices that encourage self-inquiry, such as journalling or meditation (see page 44), can help you identify which obstacles or limiting beliefs are holding you back.

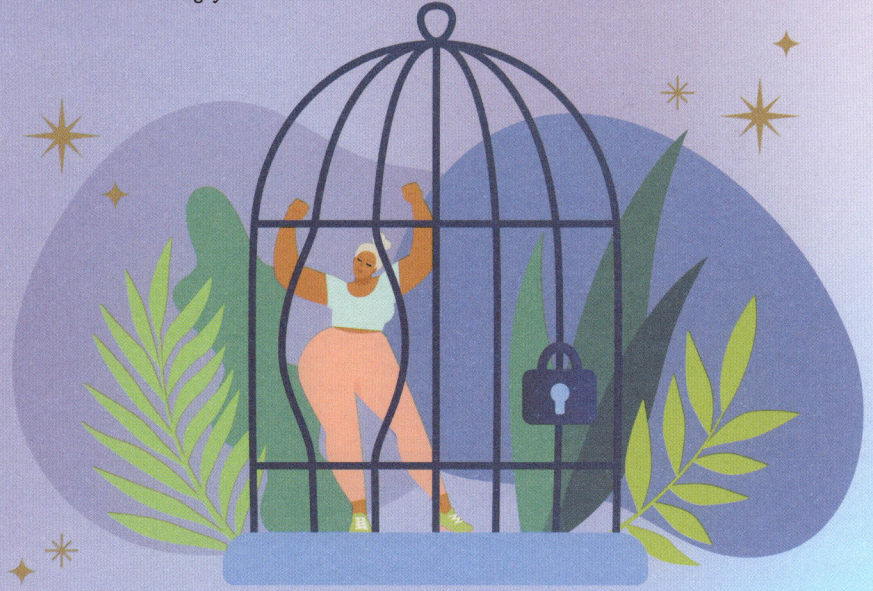

## The impact

The energy you put out shapes the reality you attract. When doubt, fear or negative beliefs take over, they create resistance, and can even manifest the very outcomes you're trying to avoid.

Manifestation works on the principle that similar things – or energies – are attracted to one another. So, positive thoughts manifest positive experiences and vice versa. Negative thought patterns can attract unhelpful energies towards you, which some people describe as 'lowering your vibrational frequency'. For example, if someone is manifesting a new job but constantly thinking "I'm not good enough", they are vibrating at the frequency of inadequacy and self-doubt. This energy could block opportunities and lead to circumstances that reinforce their anxieties.

Our subconscious minds tend to focus on what is most emotionally charged, or as the author James Redfield put it, "Energy flows where attention goes". So, if you direct a lot of energy towards negative or unhelpful thoughts – such as fear or self-doubt – you might inadvertently end up reinforcing what you were hoping to avoid.

Obstacles such as fear of failure can also result in patterns of self-sabotage. This might present as avoidance, procrastination, not putting in the necessary effort, or second-guessing opportunities. A distorted view of reality could also

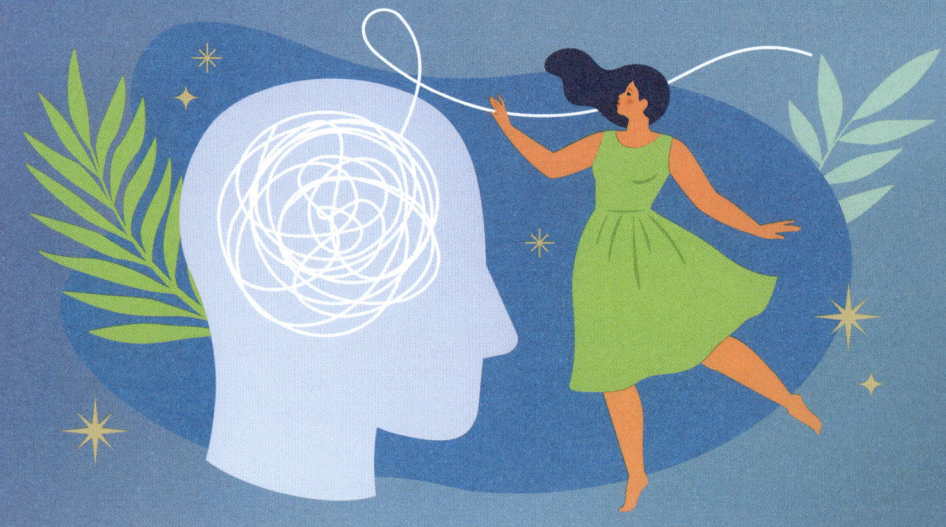

start to take hold, where you focus on potential problems or setbacks rather than possibilities and opportunities.

When we doubt, overanalyse or focus on fear, it stops us from allowing manifestations to flow. For example, someone who is manifesting financial abundance, but constantly worries about money – checking their bank account obsessively and stressing over every expense. Even though they set intentions for wealth, their energy is rooted in scarcity and fear. They are so focused on 'not having enough' that they unknowingly block opportunities for financial growth – such as a job offer or an unexpected gift. It can also leave us feeling paralysed and unable to take the next steps to achieve our goals. Without action, we can't create the conditions for manifestation to occur.

> When we doubt, overanalyse, or focus on fear, it stops us from allowing manifestations to flow

## Overcoming

Once you've identified the blocks in your manifestation practice, you can start shifting them. By reframing negative thoughts, using affirmations and engaging in deep inner work, you can replace doubt and resistance with confidence and alignment.

We can begin by using reframing techniques to help us see things differently. When our manifestations don't seem to be yielding results, instead of feeling defeated or seeing it as a catastrophe, we can instead think of it as a helpful lesson guiding us closer to our goals. For example, you could be trying to manifest a successful business, but launch a product that doesn't sell well. Instead of seeing this as a sign that you're not meant to succeed, you examine and analyse what didn't work – leading you to adjust the marketing, tweak the product, or learn more about your audience. By treating the 'failure' as valuable *feedback*, you can grow from the experience and more accurately align your actions and offerings with your ultimate vision of success.

Another powerful tool for transformation is the use of affirmations. The subconscious mind absorbs repeated thoughts as truth, so repeating

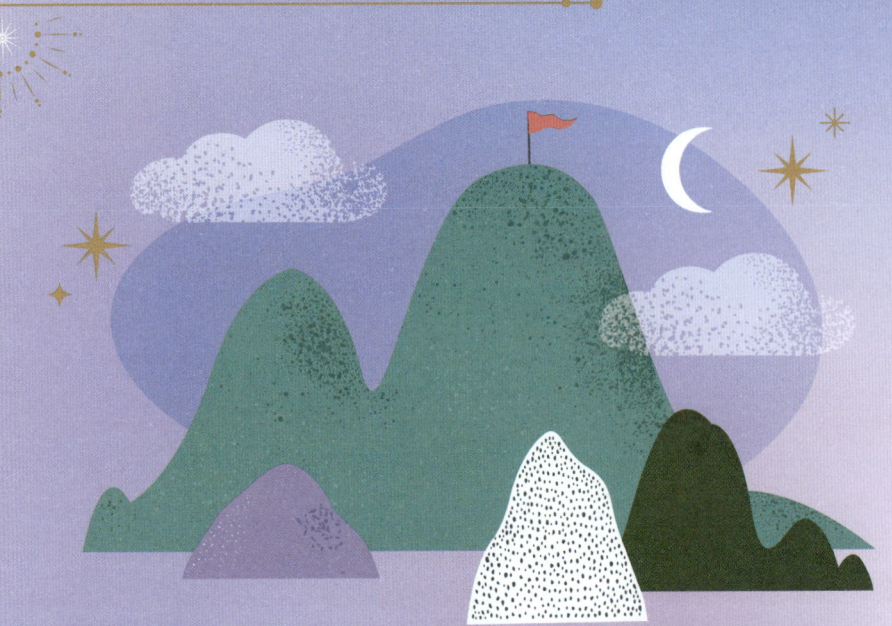

affirmations can help to reprogram negative beliefs and shift focus from self-doubt to self-empowerment. In order to create your own personalised affirmations, there are a few things to keep in mind. First, it's important to speak in the present tense – as if what you hope to be is already true, such as "I am abundant" instead of "I will be abundant". It's also useful to be specific, and really *feel* the affirmation as you say it (or write it), so that it is infused with a powerful emotional charge. Finally, consistent practice is key – as we've already discussed, some find it helpful to attach their affirmation practice to another part of their daily routine. You can use the limiting beliefs you have identified, and transform them into your own personalised positive affirmations. For example, "Money is hard to come by" changes to "Money flows to me with ease and abundance"; and "Love never works out for me" can become "I attract loving and healthy relationships effortlessly".

It could be helpful to work with a professional if you are facing deeply rooted blocks, especially if they likely stem from childhood experiences or past traumas. Whether through therapy, counselling, mentoring or coaching, it will be useful to work through the process with someone with expertise and experience. They can help provide guidance, offer new perspectives, and suggest actionable tools to overcome the things that are holding you back. Approaches such as cognitive behavioural therapy (CBT), inner child work, hypnotherapy and shadow work might be particularly helpful.

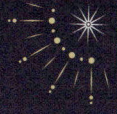

Whichever approach you choose, it's vital that you practise self-compassion and acceptance throughout. Being kind to yourself in this way will be invaluable when it comes to integrating your new learning and healing your hidden blocks. Practices like meditation and breathwork can help with this, as they encourage you to calm the mind, stay present and align energetically.

## Trusting the process

Society conditions us to expect quick results, but manifestation isn't about deadlines – it's a practice. Building resilience, cultivating growth and energetic alignment don't happen overnight. If we are overly attached to 'when' or 'how', it can create resistance instead of flow and ease.

We can look to people like Oprah Winfrey as an example of someone who successfully reframed obstacles as stepping stones rather than roadblocks. She was born into poverty and faced trauma and rejection throughout childhood and early adulthood. Despite the many hardships she faced, she persisted, and often speaks about how practising manifestation and gratitude were key to her success. In terms of overcoming blocks, we can keep this well-known Oprah quote in mind – "Challenges are gifts that force us to search for a new center of gravity. Don't fight them. Just find a new way to stand."

Just like planting a seed, manifestations require nurturing, patience and faith in order for our desired outcomes to become a reality. Sometimes what seems like delayed results might actually be 'divine timing', or the universe lining up the right people, opportunities or point in time for your desires to flourish. While identifying our blocks and putting in the work to overcome them, we need to remember that obstacles are just a part of the process. Overcoming challenges is a crucial part of progression, helping us to shift limiting beliefs and refine our vision. Every challenge you overcome brings you one step closer to your desires. Trust the journey.

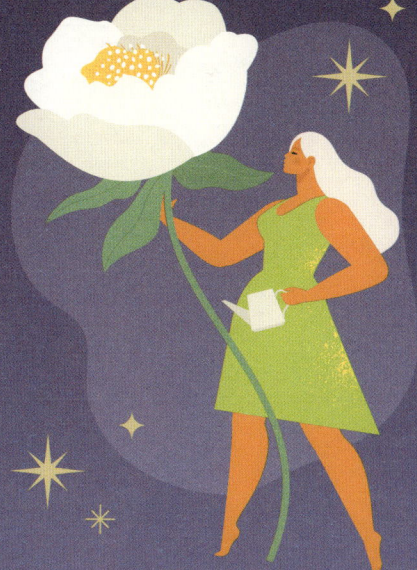

# Your manifestation goals

**GOAL SETTING IS A CORE TOOL THAT WILL SUPERCHARGE YOUR INTENTIONS TO HELP MANIFEST THE LIFE YOU WANT**

WORDS | BEATE TRIANTAFILIDIS

Setting goals for yourself comes with a wide range of benefits – if done right. Constructive goals can enhance your focus and motivation, and strengthen your sense of control. For your goals to play an effective part in your manifestation practice, first you want to be intentional about finding goals that fit you. Second, you want to calibrate them to your life at this point in time, to make sure you have the conditions in place to achieve them. Third, you embark on the practical steps towards making your goals a reality.

## Finding your goals

### Get personal

When setting goals, start with identifying your personal values. These are broader themes of what matters to you, like health, relationships, community, meaningful work and so on. Without checking in at this more fundamental level of who you are, it's easy to set goals that do not align with what matters most to you. If we do not stay anchored in our values when setting goals, we often get too influenced by what other people around us are doing or what we think we should be doing (such as a boilerplate New Year's resolution to go to the gym three times a week). To get the most benefit, your goals must be tailored to you.

## Add process-based goals

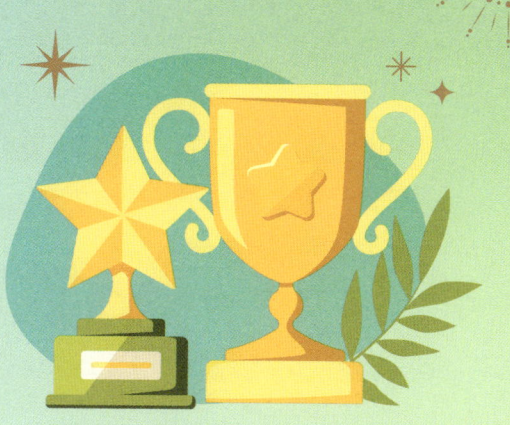

Decide on which type of goal you want to set. Typical goals are often based on the final outcome you want to achieve – for example, "Get a new job I love this year". But you can also set process-based goals, which focus on the input, or the actions you actually take towards that final goal. While process-based goals are often overlooked, they play a critical complementary role and can, for many, be more effective. In the case of the outcome-based goal of getting a new job that you love, a matching process-based goal may be spending an hour a week reviewing job openings online and submitting at least one job application every month. Process-based goals centre on actions that are in your control. Moreover, they emphasise the ongoing nature of achieving what you want. To supercharge your progress, set matching outcome-based goals and process-based goals simultaneously. They are most effective when done together. Your outcome goals show where you will end up. Your process goals set out how you get there.

## Get specific

Any goal, whether outcome-based or process-based, should be as specific as possible. If we revisit typical New Year's resolutions, they are often too general. Think "Eat healthily", "Sleep more" and "Spend less time on my phone". Specific versions of those goals may be "Eat at least five portions of fruits and vegetables every weekday", "Go to bed by 10pm every weeknight" and "Keep my phone screen time under two hours per day on average".

Specificity often implies measurability – and being able to measure and track progress towards your goals is helpful. But in the context of manifestation, creating specificity to your goals goes beyond measurement. Here, you want to consider: What will achieving my goal feel like? What will it look like? Where am I when it happens? You should be able to picture each of your goals vividly in your mind, like a scene in a movie.

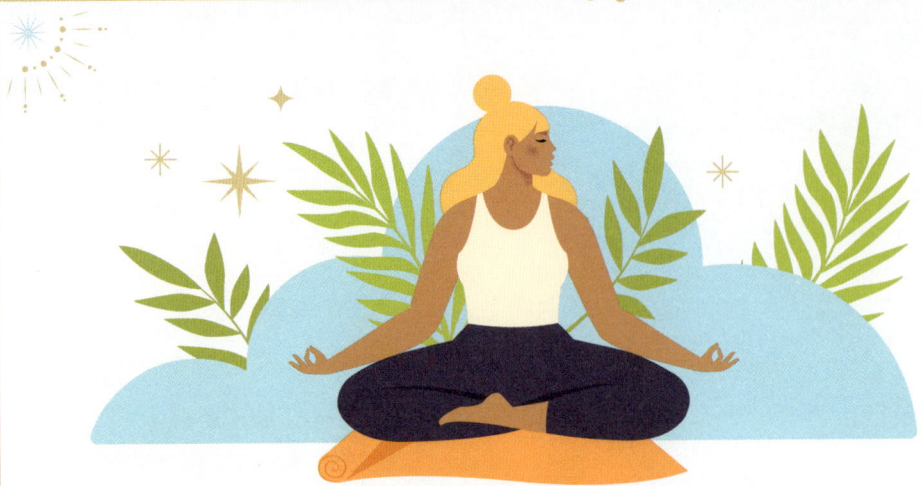

# Calibrating your goals
## Take a sense check

Once you have drafted your goals, consider them, individually and together. Do they energise and excite you? Try to tap into your immediate feelings here, rather than thinking about them intellectually. If some of them don't ignite sparks in you, take this second check: Do those goals tap into a deeper want or value rather than an immediate desire? For example, you may have a goal to call your parents every week, because you want to have a strong relationship with them, or you want to be the kind of person who is close with their parents. Goals can be centred on what kind of person you want to be, as well as activities you want to do.

## Narrow your focus

Identifying which goals you are *not* focusing on is equally as essential as setting out the goals you want to achieve. Many of us attempt to actively pursue too many goals at once. The advice on the number of goals to pursue at a given time varies, but it is likely fewer than you think. Jay Shetty – podcaster, author and life coach – recommends focusing on only one professional goal and one personal goal at a time. In the book *Slow Productivity*, productivity expert Cal Newport advocates for working on a maximum of three projects at any given time.

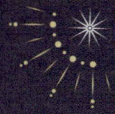

## Get real about distractions

Beyond limiting your number of goals, get clear on what is likely to distract you from them. What are the things you often say yes to that are not core priorities or linked to your top goals? What often derails our goals is typically not the things we don't want to do, but all the things we 'kind of' want to do, as Oliver Burkeman highlights in his book *Four Thousand Weeks – Time Management for Mortals*. Getting clear about your "middling priorities" is a first step to staying centred around what really matters to you. To stay on track, make this your mantra: "I can do anything, but not everything."

### Be wildly ambitious in your ultimate outcome-based goals, and conservative in your process-based goals

## Plan for non-optimal conditions

Consistency is essential when it comes to goals. For consistency to be achievable in practice, make each step towards your ultimate goals smaller than you think you need to, so that you can complete it also when life is not going exactly to plan. This is where the distinction between outcome goals and the process towards them becomes helpful. Be wildly ambitious in your ultimate outcome-based goals, and conservative in your process-based goals. Your process-based goals should be sufficiently small that you can complete them even during a non-optimal day or week or month. If you set goals that you can only manage when you feel at your best or when everything is going exactly as you hoped across all aspects of your life, you will soon find it hard to stick with them over time, as things will often not go to plan.

# Manifesting your goals

## Cement your belief with affirmations

Only when you believe that something is possible will you take the necessary steps of action towards it. Cement a belief in yourself achieving your goals by using affirmations. These are statements about something you want to be true, which you express as if they were already realised. If your ultimate goal is to get a job you love, your affirmation may be "I am doing work that I love". You can also create affirmations that assert the qualities you need to have to achieve ambitious goals more generally. Dedication, focus, patience, resilience and optimism are some qualities that may be relevant. Whatever qualities you want to cultivate, the format of the affirmations remain present-tense 'I am' statements: "I am dedicated", "I am focused", "I am patient" and so on. (Read more about affirmations on page 27.)

## Connect with the future

Alongside affirmations, imagining the future where you have achieved your goals cements the belief in them that you need to stay motivated – and it primes your brain to spot opportunities to work towards them. (For more on visualisation see page 24.) In addition to visualisation techniques, future journalling is a powerful tool here. Get your journal, pretend to be yourself in the future when you have achieved your goals, and write the story of achieving them and how it felt.

When connecting with the imagined future, make sure you imagine achieving your process-based goals as well as your final outcome-based goal. If your goal is to publish a book and your related process goal is to write every Sunday afternoon for an hour, imagine showing up at your desk every week, as well as imagining yourself proudly holding that final printed copy in your hands.

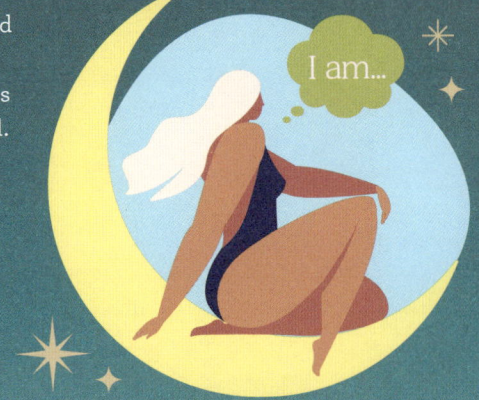

## Plan when

Now that you have your goals and have calibrated them, make a concrete plan for when you will dedicate time to work on them. Manifesting your goals requires action. Two top tips from Ali Abdaal in his book *Feel-Good Productivity* are to tag the work you will do on your goal onto an existing habit or routine (for example, meditate while your morning tea brews), and to block specific times in your schedule, just like you would with appointments with other people. In the same way that you want to plan exactly when to take action towards your goals, make a plan for when to do your affirmations and visualisations too.

## Celebrate progress

Finally, as you start manifesting your goals, celebrate every step of progress. Each time you hit one of your process-based goals, record that and acknowledge it. By doing so, you create proof for yourself that your goals are possible for you and that the future you want is within your reach.

### A note on timelines

Placing a realistic timeline on your outcome-based goals can be tricky. We typically underestimate how long it will take to achieve something. The recommendation from productivity expert Cal Newport in his book *Slow Productivity* is to take your initial time estimate and double it. For outcome-based goals where you have limited control on the timeline (for example, finding a romantic partner), consider omitting a time-bound deadline on the goal itself, and focus on sticking with your related process-based goals (for example, reaching out to at least one new person a week).

# Complementary *practices*

ENHANCE YOUR MANIFESTATION JOURNEY WITH INTERCONNECTED ACTIVITIES THAT CULTIVATE CLARITY, CREATIVITY AND ALIGNMENT

WORDS | JOSE HALL

## Creative expression

Creative expression is an innate part of being human. Whether you choose to paint, dance, write poetry, play an instrument or do something else creative, allowing yourself the space and time to express yourself can be hugely beneficial for both your manifestation practice and your general wellbeing. A state of 'creative flow' – when we are deeply immersed and focused on a creative activity – is similar to meditation; it anchors us to the present moment. As self-consciousness fades and ideas flow, there is a natural reduction in overthinking and attachment to outcomes, creating fertile ground for manifestations to unfold.

Dedicating time to creativity allows you to dream and imagine. Within this free-thinking mindset, your desires can take shape more clearly. Maybe you're doodling without an idea in mind, then look down and realise you've drawn the garden of your dreams. Whatever your outlet, creative expression can reinforce self-belief in your ability to generate desired outcomes.

# Meditation & mindfulness

Meditation is a perfect accompaniment for manifestation that anyone can access. It's about quieting the mind, and creating space amongst the stream of thoughts and distractions that so often cloud our focus or sap our energy. Once the mind is calmer, it becomes easier to hold a clear mental image of your desires. A regular meditation practice also deepens self-awareness, helping you to identify subconscious blocks and connect to your inner wisdom. By tuning in to our intuition in this way, we can ensure our manifestations truly align with our values, beliefs and needs. Meditation encourages trust in the process and a detachment from limiting thoughts, which reduces the urge to obsess over results and allows our manifestations to unfold naturally.

Mindfulness is a core aspect of meditation, helping us learn how to focus our mind on the present, observing thoughts and feelings without judgment. Honing this skill of being in the moment will make visualisations more vivid, emotionally charged, and potentially more powerful. The beauty of mindfulness is that it doesn't have to be a formal practice – it can also be applied to everyday activities such as eating, brushing your teeth, or simply walking or sitting and observing your surroundings.

Other meditation techniques to help bring clarity include choosing a focal point (such as your breath) or a mantra (such as "om", or a calming phrase) to focus on. You could also try the body scan technique, which brings attention to each part of your body, noticing any sensations or tension without attaching judgment.

# Journalling

Journalling allows us to embark on an exploration of our thoughts and feelings, which can be really helpful for identifying our core values, beliefs and desires. This kind of intentional introspection is crucial for discerning what you truly want to manifest and what might be getting in your way. Journalling can help to reinforce the positive mindset you have cultivated through manifestation, by providing a space to write down affirmations, action plans or even to energetically embody your desires by exploring your experiences of them in the present tense. When we really *feel* what we are writing, our subconscious has a harder time telling the difference between what we are actually experiencing and what we are just thinking about. Journalling can be a tool to tap in to the energetic frequency of a time when the future you're manifesting is already happening.

When you journal, you give yourself space to process emotions, gain perspective, identify patterns and release unhelpful energies that might be stopping you from achieving your goals. It is a private space where you can offload your emotions in a raw and open way, which can support you in releasing negativity and clearing energetic blocks. You can also use journalling as a tool to help keep track of your progress, stay motivated and celebrate your successes. Looking back at past entries can reinforce belief in yourself and remind you of the powerful ability you have to manifest your dreams.

# Exercise, breath & posture

Manifestation is a practice, requiring commitment and a belief in long-term results. The same is true of exercise. Physical activity improves cognitive function, which can help you stay focused and feel more inspired to make changes in your life. It also releases endorphins, natural hormones that boost mood and can even relieve pain. Exercise promotes feelings of pleasure that can enhance your general wellbeing, reduce anxiety and improve sleep – all important factors for successful manifestation practice.

You can also support a positive mind-body connection with breath work. With roots in ancient spiritual and healing practices (like Buddhism, Taoism and yoga, among others), deep, intentional breathing calms the nervous system and can influence our physical and mental wellbeing in different ways. Techniques such as box breathing (inhale, hold, exhale, hold – each for the same number of seconds) or alternate nostril breathing (taking turns to inhale and exhale through each nostril) can help to clear brain fog and improve clarity. Similarly, we can try approaches such as 'breath of fire' (a passive, gentle inhalation followed by a rapid, forceful exhalation using the diaphragm) to increase energy, confidence and attraction power.

How you hold yourself is also important. An open, upright posture helps to boost confidence and self-worth (key elements for attracting abundance), while a slouched posture is linked to self-doubt and low-energy states that we want to avoid. Try intentionally striking a power pose – stand tall, shoulders back – to help raise your energetic presence.

# Interactive *exercises*

50   IDENTIFYING YOUR DREAMS

52   WANT VS NEED

54   WHAT TYPE OF MANIFESTOR ARE YOU?

56   AFFIRMATION POWER

58   CULTIVATING AN ATTITUDE OF GRATITUDE

60   A DAY IN YOUR MANIFESTED LIFE

62   SOURCES OF STRENGTH AND SUPPORT

64   CREATING A MANIFESTATION SPACE

66   WHAT HAVE YOU ALREADY MANIFESTED?

68   MANIFESTATION BLOCKS CHECK-IN

70   WHAT SPARKS YOUR SOUL?

72   MINDSET FLOWCHART

74   MANIFESTATION MOOD BOARD

# Identifying *your* dreams

**FOR EFFECTIVE MANIFESTATION, YOU NEED CLARITY ON WHAT YOU TRULY DESIRE**

WORDS | JOSE HALL

W ithout a clear vision, your energy can become scattered, making it harder for the universe to align with your intentions. This exercise will help you define your dreams, both big and small, and distinguish between passing whims and deeply rooted goals. By getting specific about what you want, you can ensure your manifestations align with your values and passions. Take a moment to reflect deeply and write freely.

---

Which past or present experiences, achievements or possessions make you feel fulfilled?

Imagine if time, money and fear weren't obstacles
– what would you pursue?

........................................................................................................
........................................................................................................
........................................................................................................
........................................................................................................
........................................................................................................
........................................................................................................

Write yourself a brief vision statement for your ideal life.
Write as if your dreams have already become reality, emphasising how
you feel, what you do and what surrounds you in this ideal future.

........................................................................................................
........................................................................................................
........................................................................................................
........................................................................................................
........................................................................................................
........................................................................................................
........................................................................................................

Your goals may evolve over time, and that's okay. As you grow and gain new experiences, your desires, priorities and perspective might shift in unexpected ways – that's a natural part of the manifestation journey. Revisit this list periodically to check if these dreams still resonate with you. If something no longer feels right, give yourself permission to adjust your vision and set new intentions that feel more aligned.

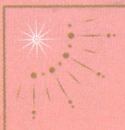
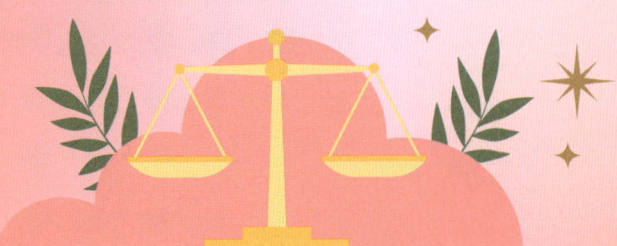

# Want vs need

**SOMETIMES, WE FOCUS ON WHAT WE WANT, RATHER THAN WHAT TRULY SERVES US**

WORDS | JOSE HALL

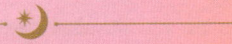

It's easy to get caught up in external desires – material success, recognition or specific outcomes – without questioning whether we actually need these things to live a fulfilled life. Often, these desires stem from societal expectations, ego or short-term gratification rather than our soul's authentic path. This exercise helps you to distinguish between surface-level wants and meaningful needs. When you focus on what genuinely nourishes your growth, happiness and purpose, manifestations become more aligned.

List three things you want to manifest in your life.

1.

2.

3.

For each thing you listed, ask yourself:
Why do I want this? How will it improve my life?

Write a sentence or two envisioning what your life looks like after receiving each of these manifestations. How does it feel?

.....................................................................................................
.....................................................................................................
.....................................................................................................
.....................................................................................................
.....................................................................................................

If you feel called to, rewrite each manifestation
in a way that serves your highest good.

1. ..................................................................................................
.....................................................................................................

2. ..................................................................................................
.....................................................................................................

3. ..................................................................................................
.....................................................................................................

Maybe you now realise that what you truly need is a sense of freedom, connection or inner peace rather than a specific job, relationship or possession. The universe often has a way of delivering what is best for you, even if it takes a different form than you expected. Learning to trust this process allows you to manifest with greater clarity, ease and alignment.

# What type of manifestor are you?

**DIFFERENT TECHNIQUES WORK FOR DIFFERENT PEOPLE – DISCOVER WHAT WORKS FOR YOU**

WORDS | JOSE HALL

Everyone manifests differently. Understanding your natural style can help you refine your practice and focus on the techniques that work best for you. This short quiz will help you to discover your strengths so you can refine your practice accordingly. To complete, simply tick the letter that best describes you.

**1. WHEN SETTING A GOAL, I:**
- A Visualise it vividly
- B Write it down in detail
- C Speak about it with belief
- D Take immediate action

**2. I FEEL MOST IN FLOW WHEN I:**
- A Meditate and imagine my desires
- B Journal and script my future
- C Use affirmations or speak my desires aloud
- D Create vision boards or physical reminders

**3. WHEN OBSTACLES ARISE, I:**
- A Trust the universe and stay positive
- B Reflect and reframe my approach in writing
- C Use affirmations to stay motivated
- D Adjust my strategy and take new action

*Stay open to experimenting, and remember that manifestation is a personal journey*

## Your results

**MOSTLY As:**
You're a Visual Manifestor. Using imagery and practising meditation come naturally to you.

**MOSTLY Bs:**
You're a Written Manifestor. For you, journalling, scripting or writing things out works best.

**MOSTLY Cs:**
You're a Spoken Manifestor. Utilising affirmations and verbalisation is where you flow with ease.

**MOSTLY Ds:**
You're an Action-Oriented Manifestor. Your natural approach is to take active steps that solidify your intentions.

**AN EVEN MIX:**
You're a combination of the relevant Manifestor types above.

There's no single 'right' way to manifest – what matters is what feels most natural and empowering for you. If your results surprised you, consider exploring new techniques to enhance your practice. You might find that combining multiple methods strengthens your manifestations. Over time, your approach may evolve as your confidence and intuition grow. Stay open to experimenting, and remember that manifestation is a personal journey – trust yourself and enjoy the process!

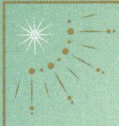

# Affirmation power

**ACKNOWLEDGE AND REFRAME YOUR LIMITING BELIEFS BY TURNING THEM INTO EMPOWERING STATEMENTS**

WORDS | JOSE HALL

Limiting beliefs are subconscious thoughts that hold you back from achieving your desires. These beliefs often stem from past experiences, societal conditioning or self-doubt. The first step to overcoming them is awareness: identifying the thoughts that limit you. The next step is transformation: replacing those negative beliefs with affirmations that support your goals. In this exercise, you'll identify a few of your own limiting beliefs and rewrite them as powerful, positive statements to shift your mindset and align your energy with your desires.

Write down one limiting belief that you hold about yourself or your ability to manifest (for example: 'I am not good enough').

Now, transform this belief into a positive affirmation. Think of creating the opposite energy to your limiting belief (for example: 'I am worthy and capable of achieving my dreams').

## Identify a few of your own limiting beliefs and rewrite them as powerful, positive statements

Limiting belief:
...................................................................................................................

Positive affirmation:
...................................................................................................................
...................................................................................................................
...................................................................................................................

Limiting belief:
...................................................................................................................

Positive affirmation:
...................................................................................................................
...................................................................................................................
...................................................................................................................

Affirmations work best when repeated consistently. Say your new statements aloud each day, write them in your journal, or place them somewhere that you will see them often. Over time, this practice will help reprogram your subconscious, replacing doubt with confidence and empowerment.

# Cultivating an attitude of gratitude

**BY FOCUSING ON WHAT YOU ALREADY APPRECIATE, YOU WILL ATTRACT MORE POSITIVITY INTO YOUR LIFE**

WORDS | JOSE HALL

Gratitude raises your vibration, attracts more abundance, and is one of the most powerful manifestation tools. Acknowledging what you already have creates an energy of fulfilment, making it easier to attract more positive experiences. Often, we focus so much on what we want that we forget to acknowledge how much we've already received. This exercise will help you to recognise the blessings in your life – both big and small – so you can cultivate a mindset of contentment and trust.

Write down five things you're grateful for in your life.

1.
2.
3.
4.
5.

Reflect on something you once wished for that is now a reality.

How does gratitude shift your perspective on your current manifestations?

Gratitude is a simple yet transformative practice. Even in challenging times, finding small moments of appreciation can help you maintain faith in your journey. The more gratitude you cultivate, the more magnetic you become to joy, success and abundance. By making gratitude a daily practice, you naturally raise your vibration and create space for more of what you desire.

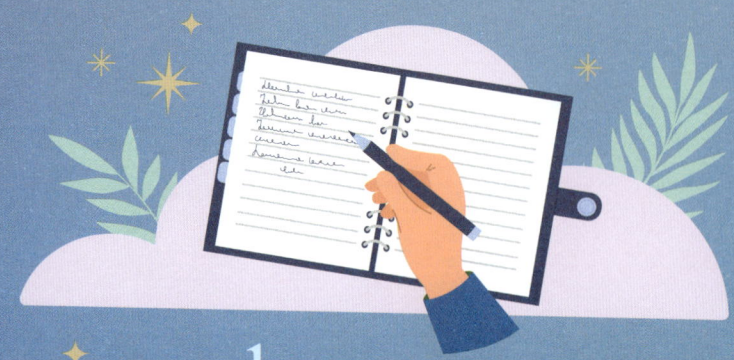

# A day *in your* manifested life

**WRITING YOUR DESIRES AS IF THEY HAVE ALREADY COME TRUE HELPS YOUR SUBCONSCIOUS ACCEPT THEM AS REALITY**

WORDS | JOSE HALL

The more vividly we connect with our desired future, the more real it becomes in our minds. This practice not only strengthens belief in your manifestations but also generates the emotions and confidence needed to attract them. In this exercise, write a journal entry from your future dream life. What does your morning look like? How do you feel as you go about your day? What achievements, relationships and experiences are part of your reality? If helpful, try meditating or visualising before writing. Or, if you naturally connect through words, just let yourself flow freely.

*Return to this exercise whenever you need a boost of motivation or to reconnect with your vision*

> Write a journal entry from the future, describing a perfect day where your dream life is already happening.

Dear diary,

Envisioning and writing about your manifested future allows you to fully immerse yourself in the emotions and experiences of your dream life. You might have surprised yourself with what flowed onto the page, revealing new desires or insights. Reading this back, you may feel inspired to refine your manifestations or adjust your affirmations. Return to this exercise whenever you need a boost of motivation or to reconnect with your vision – each time, it will become even more real.

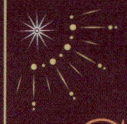

# Sources of strength and support

**ENHANCE YOUR MANIFESTATION JOURNEY BY RECOGNISING THE PEOPLE AND SUPPORT SYSTEMS THAT STRENGTHEN YOU**

WORDS | JOSE HALL

Manifesting isn't something you have to do alone. It isn't just about personal willpower – it's also about the environment and relationships that uplift and sustain you. The people, communities and even hobbies that provide encouragement, comfort and strength play a key role in helping you stay aligned with your goals. In this exercise, reflect on your sources of support, whether it's loved ones, mentors, or personal practices that ground you in times of doubt. By identifying and nurturing these connections, you create a strong foundation for your manifestation journey.

List three people – these could be friends, family, colleagues, mentors or community members – who offer you emotional or practical support. How do they uplift you?

| MY SUPPORTERS | BECAUSE... |
|---|---|
| 1. | |
| 2. | |
| 3. | |

What personal practices, hobbies or rituals help you feel strong, centred or resilient? For example: meditation, exercise, journalling, time in nature and so on.

How can you deepen your connection with these people and practices? What small action can you take to strengthen your support system?

By surrounding yourself with positive influences – both in relationships and in how you spend your time – you are creating an environment where your manifestations can flourish. Reflecting on these sources of support reminds you that you are never alone in your journey; you can draw inspiration from cherished friends and family, as well as your favourite activities. Take the time to continue nurturing these connections: reach out to a loved one, express gratitude, or make space for self-care practices that replenish your energy.

# Creating a manifestation space

**A DEDICATED SPACE FOR MANIFESTATION CAN ENHANCE FOCUS AND ALIGNMENT**

WORDS | JOSE HALL

Your environment influences your energy. Having a dedicated space can help reinforce your practice by signalling to your mind that this is a place for focus, clarity and intention setting. Designing your space to feel peaceful and inspiring can help you tap into your subconscious mind and creative energy. Even if you don't have much room to spare, a simple setup with meaningful objects can cultivate a powerful energy for manifestation.

### You can create a space that reflects where you're headed

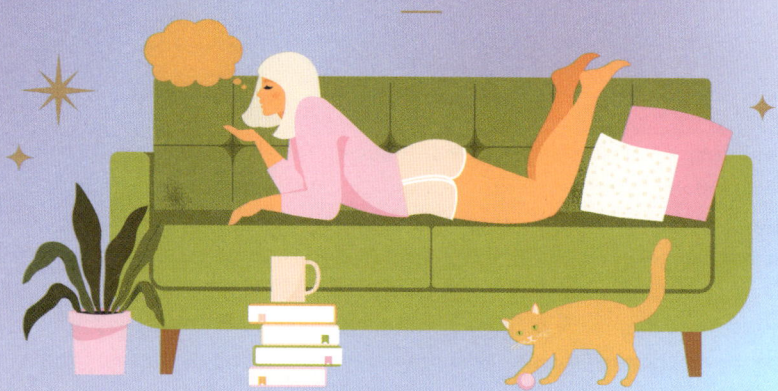

Draw or describe your ideal manifestation space.

A dedicated manifestation space serves as a physical anchor for your spiritual practice, helping you step into the energy of your desires. Even if you don't yet have your dream home or ideal surroundings, you can create a space that reflects where you're headed. If you don't have room for a physical setup right now, use this exercise as a vision-setting practice – imagining the space you will one day create as part of your manifested life.

# What have you already manifested?

**RECOGNISING PAST MANIFESTATIONS REINFORCES THE BELIEF IN YOUR POWER TO CREATE**

WORDS | JOSE HALL

Whether or not you were consciously trying to, you have already manifested many things into your life. Some may have been intentional successes, while others may have been unexpected or even undesirable. But no matter the outcome, each experience is proof of your innate ability to attract and create. Acknowledging these past manifestations reinforces your trust in the process and your own power to shape your future. Reflect on what you've already brought into your life and identify patterns in terms of how your energy, thoughts and actions contributed to those outcomes.

List three things you have already manifested – big or small, positive or negative.

1.

2.

3.

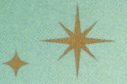

Reflect on how these things came into your life.
What energy, mindset or actions led to them?

1.

2.

3.

It's easy to overlook how much you've already accomplished and created. By taking time to recognise your past manifestations, you remind yourself that you are always shaping your reality. Use this reflection as proof that you have the power to manifest what you desire, both now and in the future.

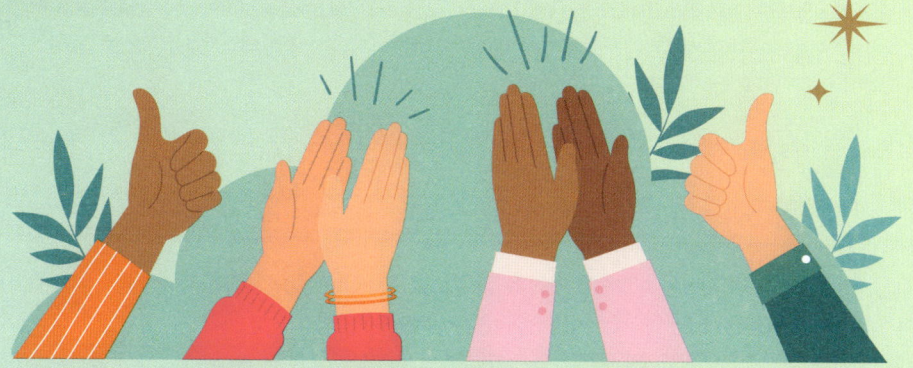

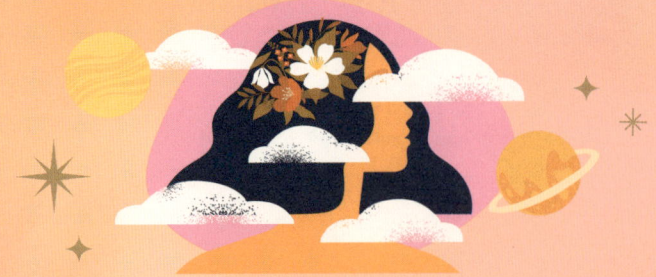

# Manifestation blocks *check-in*

**IDENTIFYING AND RELEASING BLOCKS HELPS YOU TO MANIFEST WITH GREATER EASE AND CONFIDENCE**

WORDS | JOSE HALL

Sometimes, the biggest obstacles to manifestation aren't external – they're internal. Limiting beliefs, subconscious fears and resistance can all interfere with the process, even when you're doing everything 'right'. The aim of this exercise is to help you identify what might be holding you back so you can shift your mindset and energy accordingly. Acknowledging these blocks helps you release them and replace them with more empowering beliefs. Start by reading the following common manifestation blocks, and tick off any that resonate with you:

- [ ] Fear of failure or disappointment
- [ ] Self-doubt or feelings of unworthiness
- [ ] Attachment to a specific outcome
- [ ] Impatience or lack of trust in the process
- [ ] Negative self-talk or limiting beliefs
- [ ] Focusing too much on 'how' instead of trusting the 'what'
- [ ] Resistance to change or stepping outside your comfort zone

Choose one block you want to work on. How does it show up in your life?

**BLOCK**

......................................................................................................................
......................................................................................................................

**HOW I ENCOUNTER IT**

......................................................................................................................
......................................................................................................................
......................................................................................................................
......................................................................................................................

How can you begin to release this block?
What new belief or action could replace it?

......................................................................................................................
......................................................................................................................
......................................................................................................................
......................................................................................................................
......................................................................................................................
......................................................................................................................

We all experience blocks at some point, but awareness is the first step in overcoming them. By shifting your mindset and energy, you help your manifestations to flow more easily. Releasing limiting beliefs is a process – if a particular block feels deep-rooted, be patient with yourself and consider seeking support. Keep revisiting this exercise whenever you feel stuck, and remind yourself that you are always capable of growth and transformation.

# What sparks your soul?

**DEEPEN AND ENERGISE YOUR MANIFESTATION PRACTICE BY EXPLORING WHAT IGNITES YOUR CURIOSITY AND JOY**

WORDS | JOSE HALL

Inspiration is a powerful fuel for manifestation. When you engage with things that excite and move you, you raise your energy and open yourself up to new possibilities. This exercise helps you to reflect on what truly inspires you – whether it's art, music, literature, travel, nature or certain people and experiences. By actively surrounding yourself with inspiration, you keep your mind and spirit open to fresh ideas, creative solutions and a deepened sense of purpose.

List three people who inspire you. What qualities or achievements do you admire?

| INSPIRING FIGURES | I ADMIRE THEM BECAUSE… |
|---|---|
| 1. | |
| 2. | |
| 3. | |

Name three books, films, songs or works of art that make you feel something deeply.

| INSPIRING ART | IT RESONATES WITH ME BECAUSE... |
|---|---|
| 1. | |
| 2. | |
| 3. | |

Describe a place that makes you feel most alive, creative or connected.

How can you invite more inspiration into your daily life?

Recognising and engaging with what inspires you lets you align yourself with creativity, joy and new possibilities. Inspiration and enjoyment expand your perspective, and strengthen your vision. Try to make space for inspiration daily, whether by consuming art, having meaningful conversations, or simply observing the beauty around you. The more you engage with what moves you, the more effortlessly you attract the life you desire.

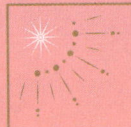

# Mindset flowchart

**IDENTIFY YOUR CURRENT MANIFESTATION FOCUS AND DISCOVER WHAT MIGHT HELP YOU MOVE FORWARD**

WORDS | JOSE HALL

Manifestation isn't a one-size-fits-all process. Sometimes we need more clarity, while other times we need to take action or practise patience. This simple flowchart will help you to identify where you are in your manifestation journey and what might help you to move forward. Answer each question honestly, and follow the path to discover your current focus area. Whether it's refining your vision, taking action, strengthening belief, or learning to let go, remember that clarity, action, belief and surrender all play essential roles in manifestation.

## Wherever you land, trust that each stage of the process is valuable

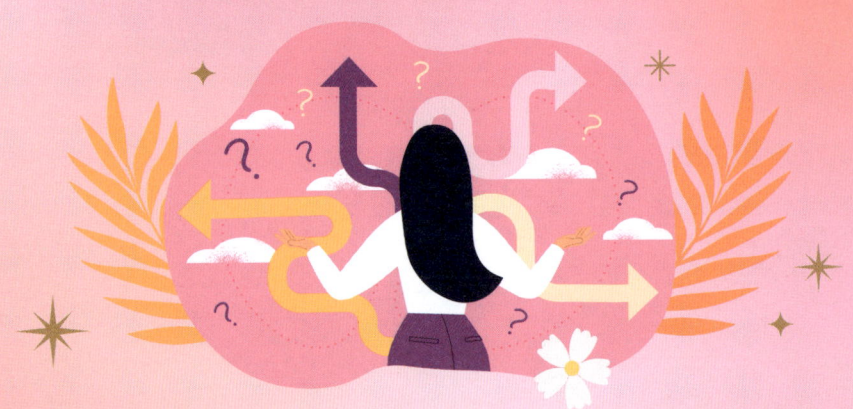

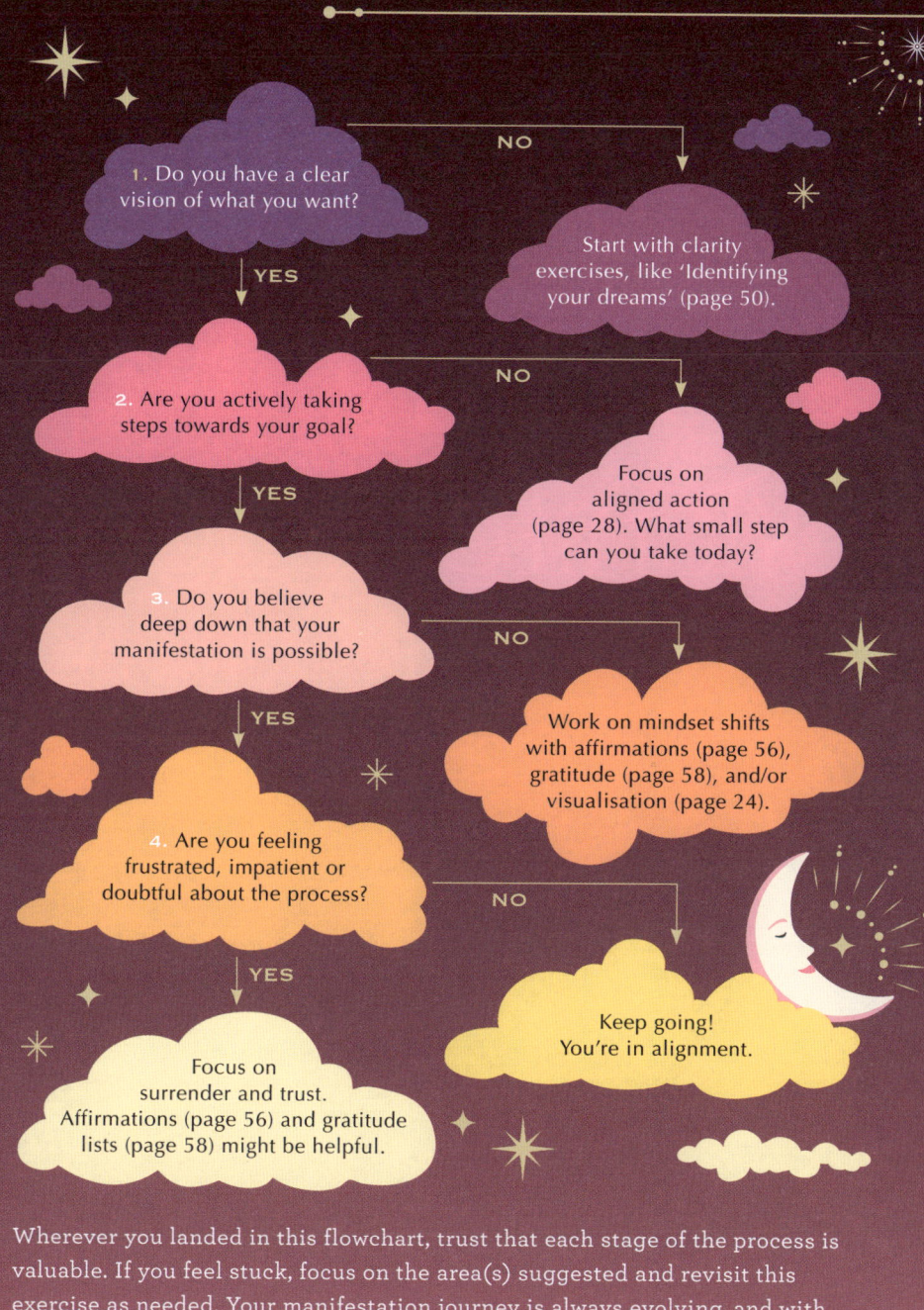

Wherever you landed in this flowchart, trust that each stage of the process is valuable. If you feel stuck, focus on the area(s) suggested and revisit this exercise as needed. Your manifestation journey is always evolving, and with each step, you're moving closer to your desires.

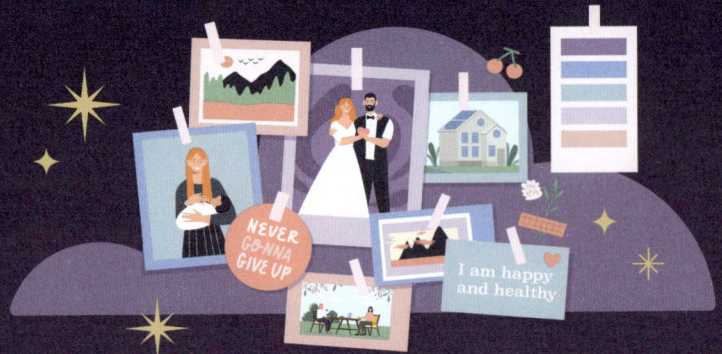

# Manifestation mood board

**A VISUAL REPRESENTATION OF YOUR DREAMS CAN MAKE THEM FEEL MORE REAL AND ATTAINABLE**

WORDS | JOSE HALL

Creating a mood board is a fun, intuitive way to connect with your desires. By selecting images, colours, words and symbols that align with your manifestations, you create a powerful visual anchor that keeps your intentions front and centre. This practice helps strengthen belief, spark inspiration, and reinforce your alignment with your desires. Whether you prefer drawing, collage-making or using digital tools, this exercise encourages you to creatively explore your dream life in a tangible way.

> Your mood board can serve as a daily reminder of your desires and the energy you are calling in

## CHOOSE YOUR BOARD

For a physical mood board, you will need a piece of card – A3 is a good starting size, but you can always use A4 and add extra sheets as required. Alternatively, you can use a digital tool if you prefer, then print out your final piece.

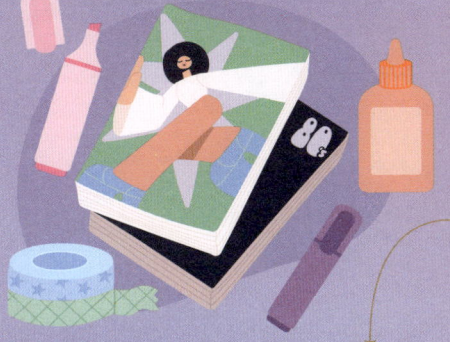

## GATHER YOUR MATERIALS

Select a variety of relevant magazines, photographs, printouts, stickers, markers and so on, as well as some tape, adhesive or glue dots to fix everything in place.

## GET CREATIVE

Create a mood board that reflects your manifested life! Consider including:

- ✦ Images that represent your desires (e.g. homes, travel, relationships, career).
- ✦ Colours, textures or symbols that evoke the emotions you want to feel.
- ✦ Affirmations, quotes or keywords that inspire and align with your vision.

*If you have space to hang it up, consider putting your finished mood board in a frame to protect it.*

Once you're happy with it, place your mood board somewhere you'll see it often. It can now serve as a daily reminder of your desires and the energy you are calling in. Spend a few moments each day looking at it, feeling into the emotions it evokes, and visualising yourself already living that reality. As your dreams evolve, or come true, you can update your board to reflect your ever-growing vision.

- 78 USING YOUR JOURNAL
- 80 PROMPT IDEAS
- 82 THE 52-WEEK DIARY
- 186 END-OF-YEAR REFLECTIONS
- 191 LOOKING TO THE FUTURE
- 192 NEXT YEAR

# Using your journal

THIS SECTION CONTAINS A YEAR'S WORTH OF WEEKLY DIARY PAGES TO HELP YOU KEEP TRACK OF YOUR MANIFESTATION PRACTICE. HERE ARE SOME TIPS ON HOW TO MAKE THE MOST OF EACH ELEMENT

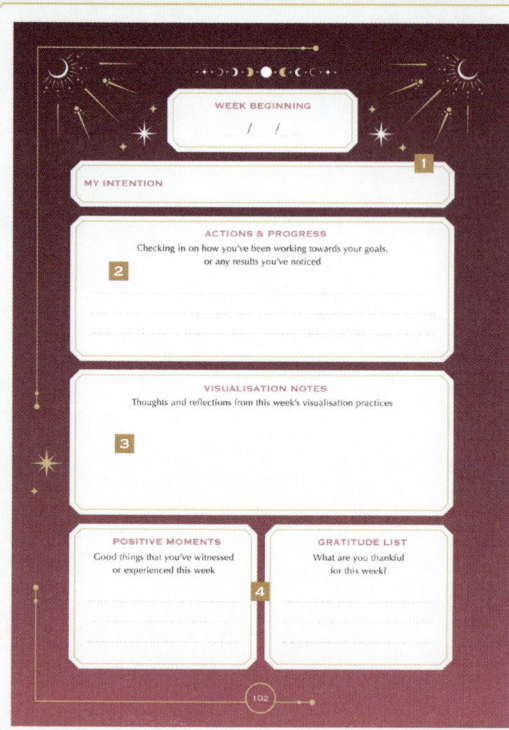

**1**

### SET YOUR INTENTION

Define your manifestation focus for the week. Make it clear, concise and specific.

**2**

### MONITOR PROGRESS

Keep track of the proactive steps you are currently taking towards your goals, as well as your overall progress and any other breakthroughs.

**3**

### VISUALISATION SPACE

Try to engage in a few moments of dedicated visualisation practice several times a week. Use this space to draw, doodle or describe what you envision.

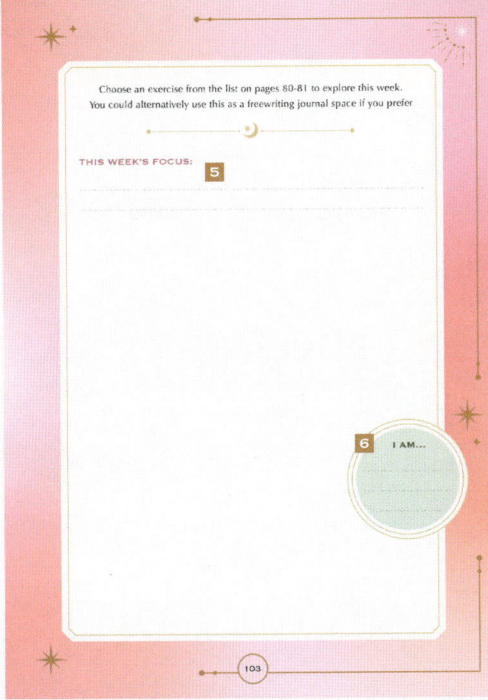

**4**

## POSITIVITY & GRATITUDE

Cultivate a positive mindset by recognising the everyday things that bring you joy. Take note of any happy moments and keep a gratitude list.

**5**

## YOUR WEEKLY FOCUS

This is a flexible space for you to curate your manifestation practice for the week. You can repeat an exercise that resonated with you from pages 50-75, choose a focus prompt to explore from the suggestions on pages 80-81 overleaf, or simply use it as a freewriting space to reflect on your manifestation journey this week.

**6**

## AFFIRMATIONS

Jot down a few 'I am…' affirmations for the week. Repeat them to yourself to cement the beliefs in your mind.

## Quarterly *check-in*

Every 13 weeks, the right-hand page will instead prompt you to imagine your future self, and write a 'Dear past me' letter. Visualise having achieved your goals, and consider what advice you would offer yourself now.

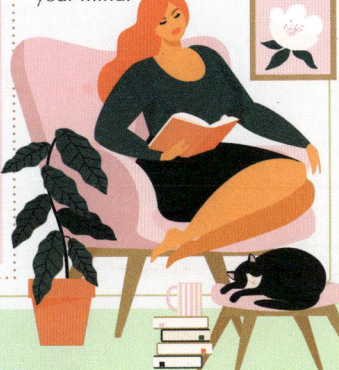

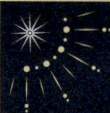
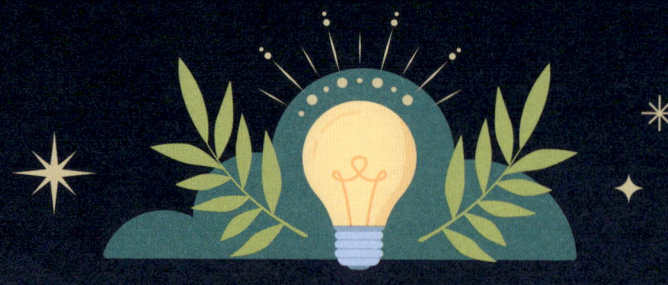

# Prompt *ideas*

✦ HERE ARE SOME SUGGESTIONS FOR TOPICS TO EXPLORE
IN YOUR WEEKLY JOURNAL FOCUS PAGE

## INTENTIONS & CLARITY

**Goals:** List your current manifestation goals. For each one, explain how they align with your lifestyle and intentions (see pages 38-43 for advice).

**Intention:** Elaborate on this week's intention. Why is this something you want to focus on? How will it improve your life?

**Your values:** Write about where you want to focus your time and energy – who and what matters most to you right now?

## GRATITUDE & JOY

**Gratitude list:** Expand on this week's gratitude list – go into more detail on why you are grateful for each entry.

**Positive moments:** Expand on this week's positive moments – what happened and why did they bring you joy?

**Sources of joy:** Write a list or create a mind map of the things that make you happy. Add as many things as you can think of.

Choose the activity you would like to focus on each week, or feel free to come up with some ideas of your own.

## VISUALISATION & CREATIVITY

**Visualisation:** Pick a specific element from your recent visualisation practice and describe or draw it in as much detail as possible.

**Explore your feelings:** Create a list or a mind map of all the emotions and sensations you experience during your recent manifestation practice.

**Happy place:** Write about or draw a specific place that brings you joy or peace, and explore the reasons why you love it.

## OBSTACLES & CHALLENGES
**Self-talk:** What negative thought patterns are currently holding you back? What techniques are you using to shift your mindset?
**Weekly challenge:** What has been challenging this week? How have you reacted?
**Life lessons:** Think of a challenge you have overcome recently – what did you learn from the experience?

*You can also pick exercises from the Interactive exercises chapter (pages 50-75) to repeat throughout the year.*

## AFFIRMATIONS & SELF-CONFIDENCE
**Empowerment:** Write down ten empowering statements about yourself and your abilities.
**Personal hero:** Think of someone you look up to. What qualities do they have that you admire, and how can you embody those characteristics in your own life?
**No fear:** What would you do if you knew you couldn't fail? How would you act differently?

## ALIGNMENT & FOCUS
**Helpful hobbies:** What activities help you feel aligned with your goals, and why?
**Bringing balance:** How balanced do you feel this week? What steps can you take to redress any misalignment?
**Mindset:** Reflect on your mindset and worldview now compared to the start of your manifestation journey. How has it changed, and what impact has this had on your everyday life?

## PREPARATION & ACTION
**Make a plan:** Consider one of your manifestation goals, and make a list of the practical steps you can take to achieve it.
**Changing course:** What actions towards your goals have you had to change or reassess during your practice so far? What changes did you make and why?
**Plan B:** Do you have goals that can be accomplished by various means? Consider what alternative tactics you could try if your Plan A doesn't lead to the intended result.

## PROGRESS & SUCCESSES
**Making progress:** Elaborate on the actions you took towards your goals this week.
**Affirmation:** Which 'I am' affirmation has been the most effective in your practice so far? How has it helped shift your thought patterns?
**Recognising success:** Think about something specific you have manifested recently, and identify the steps you took to make it happen.

## THE FUTURE
**Short-term goals:** What are three things you want to achieve by the end of this year? What steps are you taking to accomplish them?
**Long-term goals:** What are three things you want to achieve in the next five to ten years? What steps can you start taking now to help you get there?
**Legacy:** How do you want people to remember you at this point in your life? What can you do today to leave a positive impact?

**WEEK BEGINNING**

....... / ....... / .......

**MY INTENTION**

**ACTIONS & PROGRESS**

Checking in on how you've been working towards your goals,
or any results you've noticed

**VISUALISATION NOTES**

Thoughts and reflections from this week's visualisation practices

**POSITIVE MOMENTS**

Good things that you've witnessed
or experienced this week

**GRATITUDE LIST**

What are you thankful
for this week?

Choose an exercise from the list on pages 80-81 to explore this week.
You could alternatively use this as a freewriting journal space if you prefer

**THIS WEEK'S FOCUS:**

I AM...

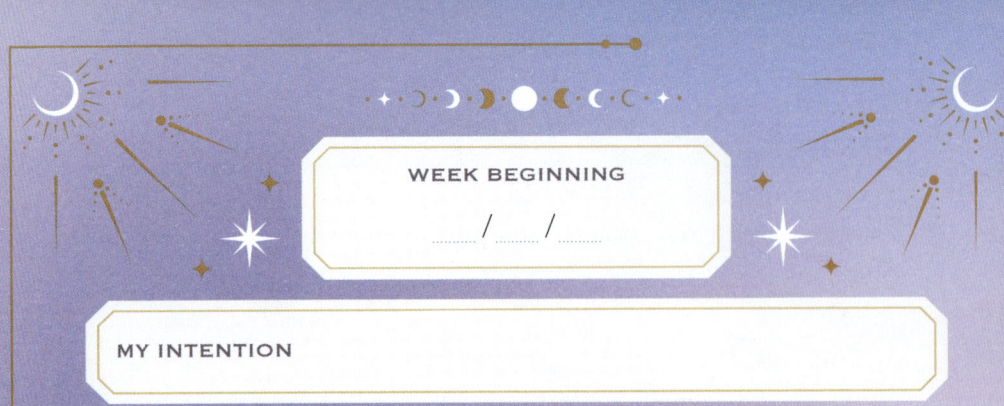

### WEEK BEGINNING

..... / ..... / .....

**MY INTENTION**

### ACTIONS & PROGRESS

Checking in on how you've been working towards your goals, or any results you've noticed

### VISUALISATION NOTES

Thoughts and reflections from this week's visualisation practices

### POSITIVE MOMENTS

Good things that you've witnessed or experienced this week

### GRATITUDE LIST

What are you thankful for this week?

Choose an exercise from the list on pages 80-81 to explore this week.
You could alternatively use this as a freewriting journal space if you prefer

**THIS WEEK'S FOCUS:**

I AM...

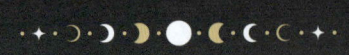

### WEEK BEGINNING

......... / ......... / .........

**MY INTENTION**

### ACTIONS & PROGRESS
Checking in on how you've been working towards your goals,
or any results you've noticed

### VISUALISATION NOTES
Thoughts and reflections from this week's visualisation practices

### POSITIVE MOMENTS
Good things that you've witnessed
or experienced this week

### GRATITUDE LIST
What are you thankful
for this week?

Choose an exercise from the list on pages 80-81 to explore this week.
You could alternatively use this as a freewriting journal space if you prefer

**THIS WEEK'S FOCUS:**

I AM...

## WEEK BEGINNING

...... / ...... / ......

## MY INTENTION

### ACTIONS & PROGRESS

Checking in on how you've been working towards your goals, or any results you've noticed

### VISUALISATION NOTES

Thoughts and reflections from this week's visualisation practices

### POSITIVE MOMENTS

Good things that you've witnessed or experienced this week

### GRATITUDE LIST

What are you thankful for this week?

Choose an exercise from the list on pages 80-81 to explore this week.
You could alternatively use this as a freewriting journal space if you prefer

**THIS WEEK'S FOCUS:**

...................................................................................................................................

...................................................................................................................................

I AM...

**WEEK BEGINNING**

......... / ......... / .........

**MY INTENTION**

### ACTIONS & PROGRESS

Checking in on how you've been working towards your goals, or any results you've noticed

### VISUALISATION NOTES

Thoughts and reflections from this week's visualisation practices

### POSITIVE MOMENTS

Good things that you've witnessed or experienced this week

### GRATITUDE LIST

What are you thankful for this week?

Choose an exercise from the list on pages 80-81 to explore this week.
You could alternatively use this as a freewriting journal space if you prefer

**THIS WEEK'S FOCUS:**
.................................................................................
.................................................................................

I AM...

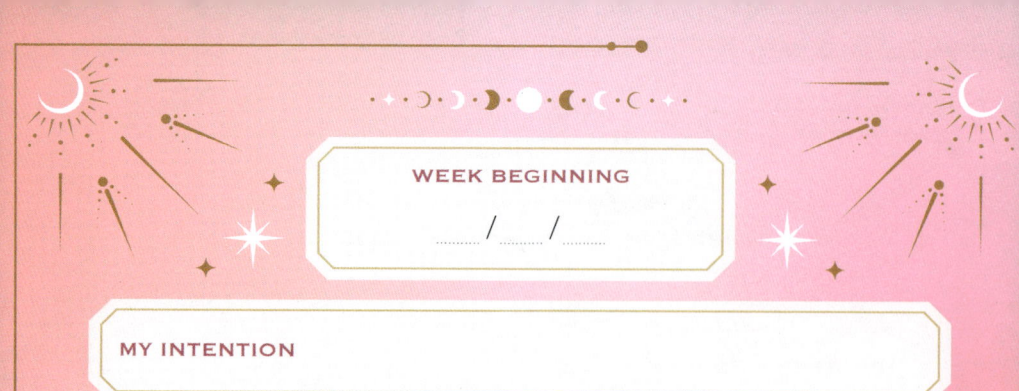

**WEEK BEGINNING**

......... / ......... / .........

**MY INTENTION**

**ACTIONS & PROGRESS**

Checking in on how you've been working towards your goals, or any results you've noticed

**VISUALISATION NOTES**

Thoughts and reflections from this week's visualisation practices

**POSITIVE MOMENTS**

Good things that you've witnessed or experienced this week

**GRATITUDE LIST**

What are you thankful for this week?

Choose an exercise from the list on pages 80-81 to explore this week.
You could alternatively use this as a freewriting journal space if you prefer

**THIS WEEK'S FOCUS:**

........................................................................................................................

........................................................................................................................

I AM...

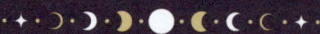

**WEEK BEGINNING**

......... / ......... / .........

**MY INTENTION**

### ACTIONS & PROGRESS

Checking in on how you've been working towards your goals, or any results you've noticed

### VISUALISATION NOTES

Thoughts and reflections from this week's visualisation practices

### POSITIVE MOMENTS

Good things that you've witnessed or experienced this week

### GRATITUDE LIST

What are you thankful for this week?

Choose an exercise from the list on pages 80-81 to explore this week.
You could alternatively use this as a freewriting journal space if you prefer

**THIS WEEK'S FOCUS:**

I AM...

### WEEK BEGINNING

......... / ......... / .........

**MY INTENTION**

### ACTIONS & PROGRESS

Checking in on how you've been working towards your goals, or any results you've noticed

### VISUALISATION NOTES

Thoughts and reflections from this week's visualisation practices

### POSITIVE MOMENTS

Good things that you've witnessed or experienced this week

### GRATITUDE LIST

What are you thankful for this week?

Choose an exercise from the list on pages 80-81 to explore this week.
You could alternatively use this as a freewriting journal space if you prefer

**THIS WEEK'S FOCUS:**

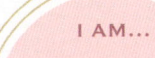

I AM...

**WEEK BEGINNING**

...... / ...... / ......

**MY INTENTION**

**ACTIONS & PROGRESS**

Checking in on how you've been working towards your goals, or any results you've noticed

**VISUALISATION NOTES**

Thoughts and reflections from this week's visualisation practices

**POSITIVE MOMENTS**

Good things that you've witnessed or experienced this week

**GRATITUDE LIST**

What are you thankful for this week?

Choose an exercise from the list on pages 80-81 to explore this week.
You could alternatively use this as a freewriting journal space if you prefer

**THIS WEEK'S FOCUS:**

................................................................

................................................................

I AM...

## WEEK BEGINNING

......... / ......... / .........

## MY INTENTION

### ACTIONS & PROGRESS
Checking in on how you've been working towards your goals, or any results you've noticed

### VISUALISATION NOTES
Thoughts and reflections from this week's visualisation practices

### POSITIVE MOMENTS
Good things that you've witnessed or experienced this week

### GRATITUDE LIST
What are you thankful for this week?

Choose an exercise from the list on pages 80-81 to explore this week.
You could alternatively use this as a freewriting journal space if you prefer

**THIS WEEK'S FOCUS:**

I AM...

### WEEK BEGINNING
......... / ......... / .........

### MY INTENTION

### ACTIONS & PROGRESS
Checking in on how you've been working towards your goals, or any results you've noticed

### VISUALISATION NOTES
Thoughts and reflections from this week's visualisation practices

### POSITIVE MOMENTS
Good things that you've witnessed or experienced this week

### GRATITUDE LIST
What are you thankful for this week?

Choose an exercise from the list on pages 80-81 to explore this week.
You could alternatively use this as a freewriting journal space if you prefer

**THIS WEEK'S FOCUS:**

..................................................................................................................

..................................................................................................................

**I AM...**

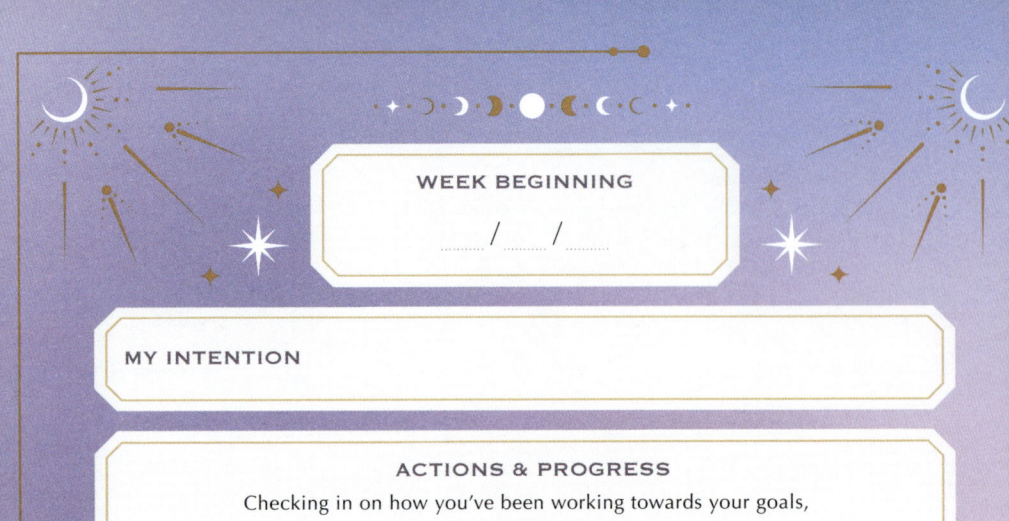

**WEEK BEGINNING**

...... / ...... / ......

**MY INTENTION**

**ACTIONS & PROGRESS**

Checking in on how you've been working towards your goals,
or any results you've noticed

**VISUALISATION NOTES**

Thoughts and reflections from this week's visualisation practices

**POSITIVE MOMENTS**

Good things that you've witnessed
or experienced this week

**GRATITUDE LIST**

What are you thankful
for this week?

Choose an exercise from the list on pages 80-81 to explore this week.
You could alternatively use this as a freewriting journal space if you prefer

**THIS WEEK'S FOCUS:**

..................................................................................................................

..................................................................................................................

I AM...

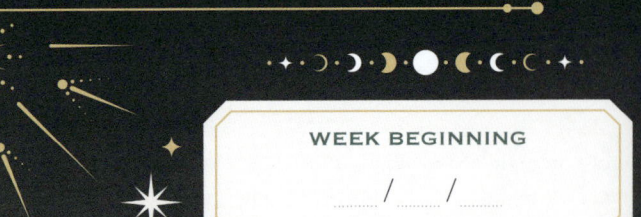

**WEEK BEGINNING**

........ / ........ / ........

**MY INTENTION**

**ACTIONS & PROGRESS**

Checking in on how you've been working towards your goals,
or any results you've noticed

**VISUALISATION NOTES**

Thoughts and reflections from this week's visualisation practices

**POSITIVE MOMENTS**

Good things that you've witnessed
or experienced this week

**GRATITUDE LIST**

What are you thankful
for this week?

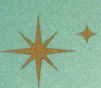

Visualise your future self who has achieved your goals, and write a letter from this perspective. Envisage that version of you and describe your future life – really focusing on your feelings. Consider what advice you'd share and what support and encouragement you would offer yourself at this point in your manifestation journey

**DEAR PAST ME,**

I AM…

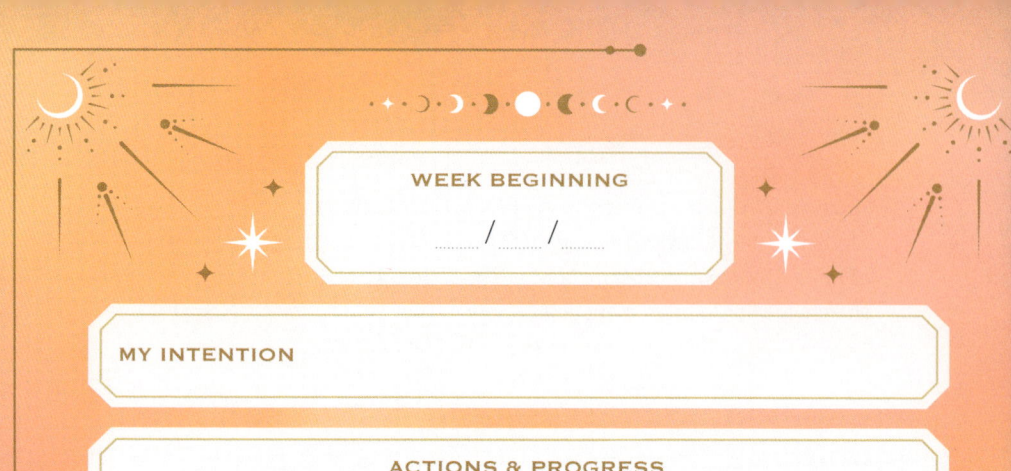

**WEEK BEGINNING**

......... / ......... / .........

**MY INTENTION**

**ACTIONS & PROGRESS**

Checking in on how you've been working towards your goals, or any results you've noticed

**VISUALISATION NOTES**

Thoughts and reflections from this week's visualisation practices

**POSITIVE MOMENTS**

Good things that you've witnessed or experienced this week

**GRATITUDE LIST**

What are you thankful for this week?

Choose an exercise from the list on pages 80-81 to explore this week.
You could alternatively use this as a freewriting journal space if you prefer

**THIS WEEK'S FOCUS:**

I AM...

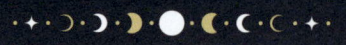

## WEEK BEGINNING

........ / ........ / ........

**MY INTENTION**

### ACTIONS & PROGRESS

Checking in on how you've been working towards your goals, or any results you've noticed

...........................................................................................................................

...........................................................................................................................

...........................................................................................................................

### VISUALISATION NOTES

Thoughts and reflections from this week's visualisation practices

### POSITIVE MOMENTS

Good things that you've witnessed or experienced this week

............................................

............................................

............................................

### GRATITUDE LIST

What are you thankful for this week?

............................................

............................................

............................................

Choose an exercise from the list on pages 80-81 to explore this week.
You could alternatively use this as a freewriting journal space if you prefer

**THIS WEEK'S FOCUS:**

I AM...

**WEEK BEGINNING**

...... / ...... / ......

**MY INTENTION**

**ACTIONS & PROGRESS**

Checking in on how you've been working towards your goals, or any results you've noticed

**VISUALISATION NOTES**

Thoughts and reflections from this week's visualisation practices

**POSITIVE MOMENTS**

Good things that you've witnessed or experienced this week

**GRATITUDE LIST**

What are you thankful for this week?

Choose an exercise from the list on pages 80-81 to explore this week.
You could alternatively use this as a freewriting journal space if you prefer

**THIS WEEK'S FOCUS:**

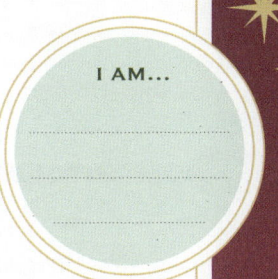

I AM...

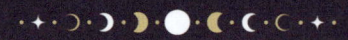

**WEEK BEGINNING**

......... / ......... / .........

**MY INTENTION**

**ACTIONS & PROGRESS**

Checking in on how you've been working towards your goals,
or any results you've noticed

**VISUALISATION NOTES**

Thoughts and reflections from this week's visualisation practices

**POSITIVE MOMENTS**

Good things that you've witnessed
or experienced this week

**GRATITUDE LIST**

What are you thankful
for this week?

Choose an exercise from the list on pages 80-81 to explore this week.
You could alternatively use this as a freewriting journal space if you prefer

**THIS WEEK'S FOCUS:**

I AM...

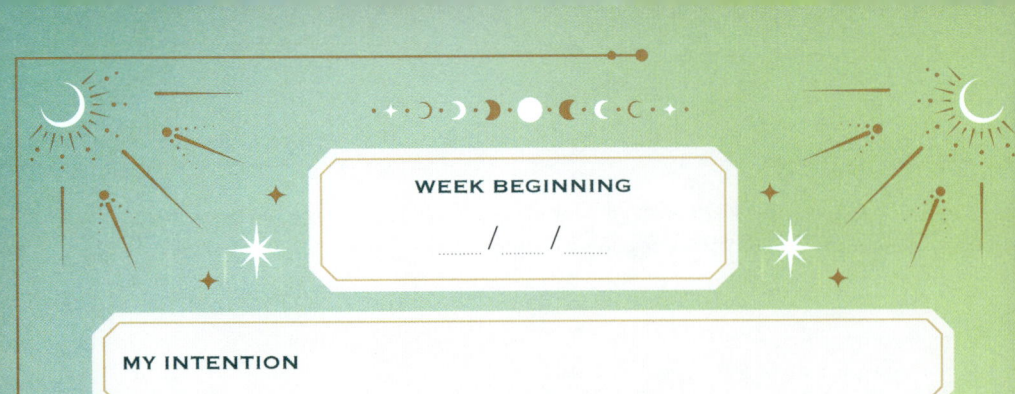

**WEEK BEGINNING**

......... / ......... / .........

**MY INTENTION**

**ACTIONS & PROGRESS**

Checking in on how you've been working towards your goals, or any results you've noticed

**VISUALISATION NOTES**

Thoughts and reflections from this week's visualisation practices

**POSITIVE MOMENTS**

Good things that you've witnessed or experienced this week

**GRATITUDE LIST**

What are you thankful for this week?

Choose an exercise from the list on pages 80-81 to explore this week.
You could alternatively use this as a freewriting journal space if you prefer

**THIS WEEK'S FOCUS:**

........................................................................................................................

........................................................................................................................

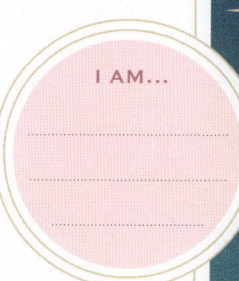

I AM...

........................................

........................................

........................................

### WEEK BEGINNING

...... / ...... / ......

**MY INTENTION**

### ACTIONS & PROGRESS

Checking in on how you've been working towards your goals, or any results you've noticed

### VISUALISATION NOTES

Thoughts and reflections from this week's visualisation practices

### POSITIVE MOMENTS

Good things that you've witnessed or experienced this week

### GRATITUDE LIST

What are you thankful for this week?

Choose an exercise from the list on pages 80-81 to explore this week.
You could alternatively use this as a freewriting journal space if you prefer

**THIS WEEK'S FOCUS:**

I AM...

**WEEK BEGINNING**

...... / ...... / ......

**MY INTENTION**

## ACTIONS & PROGRESS

Checking in on how you've been working towards your goals, or any results you've noticed

## VISUALISATION NOTES

Thoughts and reflections from this week's visualisation practices

## POSITIVE MOMENTS

Good things that you've witnessed or experienced this week

## GRATITUDE LIST

What are you thankful for this week?

Choose an exercise from the list on pages 80-81 to explore this week.
You could alternatively use this as a freewriting journal space if you prefer

**THIS WEEK'S FOCUS:**

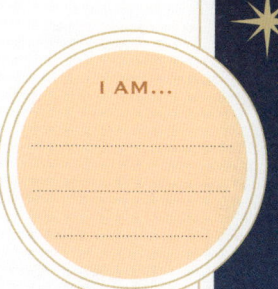

I AM...

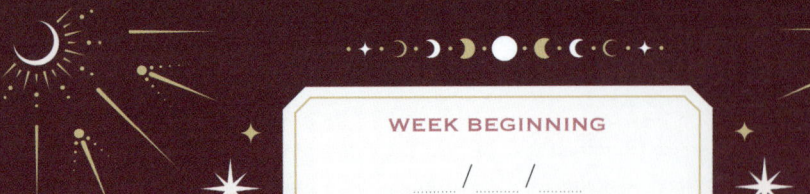

### WEEK BEGINNING

......... / ......... / .........

**MY INTENTION**

### ACTIONS & PROGRESS
Checking in on how you've been working towards your goals,
or any results you've noticed

### VISUALISATION NOTES
Thoughts and reflections from this week's visualisation practices

### POSITIVE MOMENTS
Good things that you've witnessed
or experienced this week

### GRATITUDE LIST
What are you thankful
for this week?

Choose an exercise from the list on pages 80-81 to explore this week.
You could alternatively use this as a freewriting journal space if you prefer

**THIS WEEK'S FOCUS:**

I AM...

**WEEK BEGINNING**

..... / ..... / .....

**MY INTENTION**

**ACTIONS & PROGRESS**

Checking in on how you've been working towards your goals, or any results you've noticed

**VISUALISATION NOTES**

Thoughts and reflections from this week's visualisation practices

**POSITIVE MOMENTS**

Good things that you've witnessed or experienced this week

**GRATITUDE LIST**

What are you thankful for this week?

Choose an exercise from the list on pages 80-81 to explore this week.
You could alternatively use this as a freewriting journal space if you prefer

**THIS WEEK'S FOCUS:**

I AM...

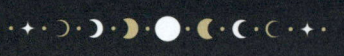

**WEEK BEGINNING**

......... / ......... / .........

**MY INTENTION**

**ACTIONS & PROGRESS**

Checking in on how you've been working towards your goals,
or any results you've noticed

**VISUALISATION NOTES**

Thoughts and reflections from this week's visualisation practices

**POSITIVE MOMENTS**

Good things that you've witnessed
or experienced this week

**GRATITUDE LIST**

What are you thankful
for this week?

Choose an exercise from the list on pages 80-81 to explore this week.
You could alternatively use this as a freewriting journal space if you prefer

**THIS WEEK'S FOCUS:**

I AM...

**WEEK BEGINNING**

...... / ...... / ......

**MY INTENTION**

**ACTIONS & PROGRESS**

Checking in on how you've been working towards your goals, or any results you've noticed

**VISUALISATION NOTES**

Thoughts and reflections from this week's visualisation practices

**POSITIVE MOMENTS**

Good things that you've witnessed or experienced this week

**GRATITUDE LIST**

What are you thankful for this week?

Choose an exercise from the list on pages 80-81 to explore this week.
You could alternatively use this as a freewriting journal space if you prefer

**THIS WEEK'S FOCUS:**

I AM...

## WEEK BEGINNING

......... / ......... / .........

**MY INTENTION**

### ACTIONS & PROGRESS
Checking in on how you've been working towards your goals, or any results you've noticed

### VISUALISATION NOTES
Thoughts and reflections from this week's visualisation practices

### POSITIVE MOMENTS
Good things that you've witnessed or experienced this week

### GRATITUDE LIST
What are you thankful for this week?

Choose an exercise from the list on pages 80-81 to explore this week.
You could alternatively use this as a freewriting journal space if you prefer

**THIS WEEK'S FOCUS:**

...........................................................................................................................

...........................................................................................................................

I AM...

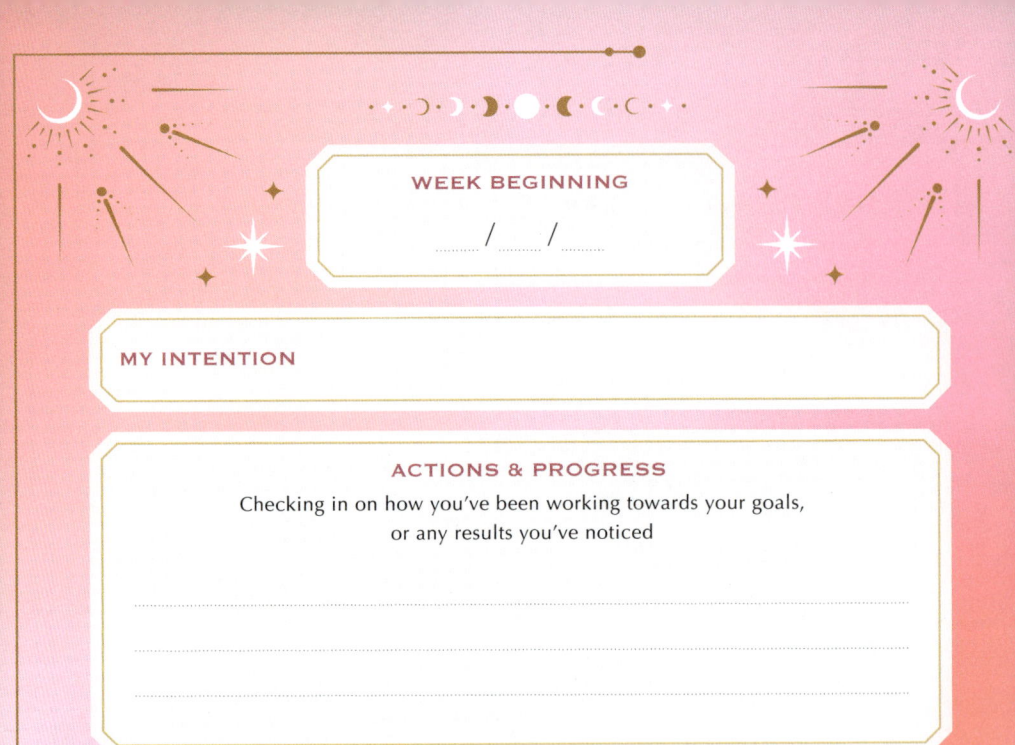

## WEEK BEGINNING

......... / ......... / .........

### MY INTENTION

### ACTIONS & PROGRESS

Checking in on how you've been working towards your goals, or any results you've noticed

### VISUALISATION NOTES

Thoughts and reflections from this week's visualisation practices

### POSITIVE MOMENTS

Good things that you've witnessed or experienced this week

### GRATITUDE LIST

What are you thankful for this week?

Visualise your future self who has achieved your goals, and write a letter from this perspective. Envisage that version of you and describe your future life – really focusing on your feelings. Consider what advice you'd share and what support and encouragement you would offer yourself at this point in your manifestation journey

**DEAR PAST ME,**

I AM…

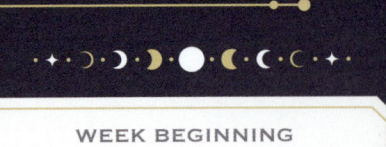

**WEEK BEGINNING**

......... / ......... / .........

**MY INTENTION**

**ACTIONS & PROGRESS**

Checking in on how you've been working towards your goals,
or any results you've noticed

**VISUALISATION NOTES**

Thoughts and reflections from this week's visualisation practices

**POSITIVE MOMENTS**

Good things that you've witnessed
or experienced this week

**GRATITUDE LIST**

What are you thankful
for this week?

Choose an exercise from the list on pages 80-81 to explore this week.
You could alternatively use this as a freewriting journal space if you prefer

**THIS WEEK'S FOCUS:**

........................................................................................................................

........................................................................................................................

I AM...

........................................

........................................

........................................

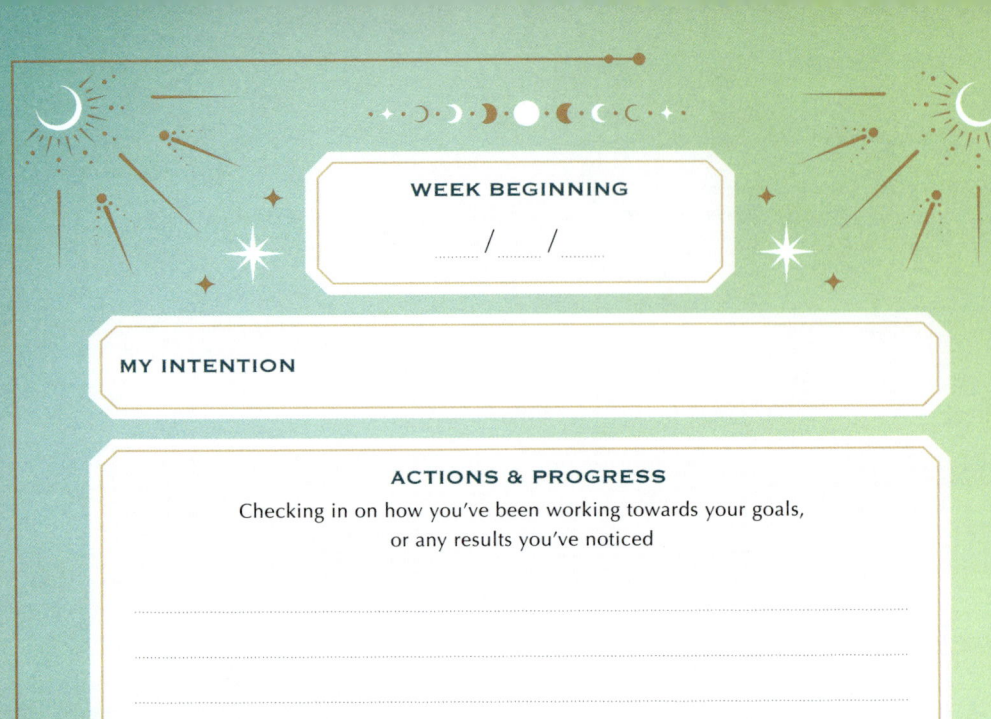

**WEEK BEGINNING**
...... / ...... / ......

**MY INTENTION**

**ACTIONS & PROGRESS**
Checking in on how you've been working towards your goals, or any results you've noticed

**VISUALISATION NOTES**
Thoughts and reflections from this week's visualisation practices

**POSITIVE MOMENTS**
Good things that you've witnessed or experienced this week

**GRATITUDE LIST**
What are you thankful for this week?

Choose an exercise from the list on pages 80-81 to explore this week.
You could alternatively use this as a freewriting journal space if you prefer

**THIS WEEK'S FOCUS:**

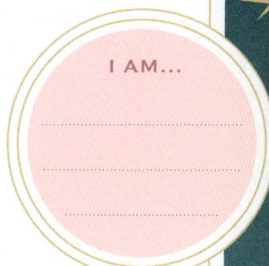

I AM...

## WEEK BEGINNING

......... / ......... / .........

### MY INTENTION

### ACTIONS & PROGRESS
Checking in on how you've been working towards your goals, or any results you've noticed

### VISUALISATION NOTES
Thoughts and reflections from this week's visualisation practices

### POSITIVE MOMENTS
Good things that you've witnessed or experienced this week

### GRATITUDE LIST
What are you thankful for this week?

Choose an exercise from the list on pages 80-81 to explore this week.
You could alternatively use this as a freewriting journal space if you prefer

**THIS WEEK'S FOCUS:**

**I AM...**

## WEEK BEGINNING

..... / ..... / .....

## MY INTENTION

### ACTIONS & PROGRESS
Checking in on how you've been working towards your goals, or any results you've noticed

### VISUALISATION NOTES
Thoughts and reflections from this week's visualisation practices

### POSITIVE MOMENTS
Good things that you've witnessed or experienced this week

### GRATITUDE LIST
What are you thankful for this week?

Choose an exercise from the list on pages 80-81 to explore this week.
You could alternatively use this as a freewriting journal space if you prefer

**THIS WEEK'S FOCUS:**

I AM…

### WEEK BEGINNING

...... / ...... / ......

**MY INTENTION**

### ACTIONS & PROGRESS

Checking in on how you've been working towards your goals, or any results you've noticed

### VISUALISATION NOTES

Thoughts and reflections from this week's visualisation practices

### POSITIVE MOMENTS

Good things that you've witnessed or experienced this week

### GRATITUDE LIST

What are you thankful for this week?

Choose an exercise from the list on pages 80-81 to explore this week.
You could alternatively use this as a freewriting journal space if you prefer

**THIS WEEK'S FOCUS:**

**I AM...**

## WEEK BEGINNING

...... / ...... / ......

## MY INTENTION

## ACTIONS & PROGRESS

Checking in on how you've been working towards your goals, or any results you've noticed

## VISUALISATION NOTES

Thoughts and reflections from this week's visualisation practices

## POSITIVE MOMENTS

Good things that you've witnessed or experienced this week

## GRATITUDE LIST

What are you thankful for this week?

Choose an exercise from the list on pages 80-81 to explore this week.
You could alternatively use this as a freewriting journal space if you prefer

**THIS WEEK'S FOCUS:**

I AM...

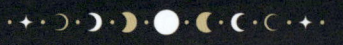

## WEEK BEGINNING

........... / ........... / ...........

**MY INTENTION**

### ACTIONS & PROGRESS
Checking in on how you've been working towards your goals, or any results you've noticed

### VISUALISATION NOTES
Thoughts and reflections from this week's visualisation practices

### POSITIVE MOMENTS
Good things that you've witnessed or experienced this week

### GRATITUDE LIST
What are you thankful for this week?

Choose an exercise from the list on pages 80-81 to explore this week.
You could alternatively use this as a freewriting journal space if you prefer

**THIS WEEK'S FOCUS:**

I AM...

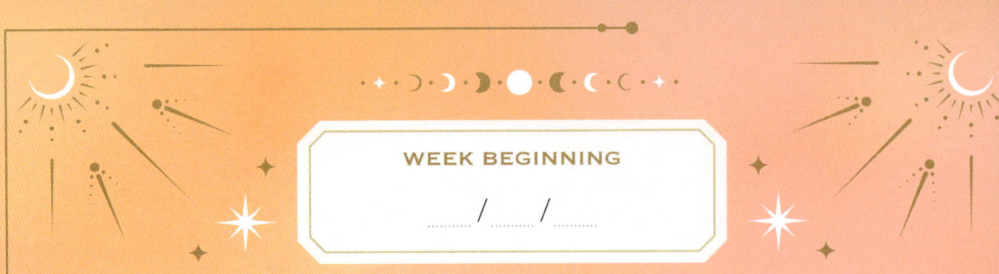

## WEEK BEGINNING

......... / ......... / .........

## MY INTENTION

## ACTIONS & PROGRESS

Checking in on how you've been working towards your goals, or any results you've noticed

## VISUALISATION NOTES

Thoughts and reflections from this week's visualisation practices

## POSITIVE MOMENTS

Good things that you've witnessed or experienced this week

## GRATITUDE LIST

What are you thankful for this week?

Choose an exercise from the list on pages 80-81 to explore this week.
You could alternatively use this as a freewriting journal space if you prefer

**THIS WEEK'S FOCUS:**

I AM...

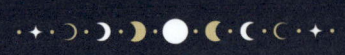

## WEEK BEGINNING

......... / ......... / .........

**MY INTENTION**

### ACTIONS & PROGRESS

Checking in on how you've been working towards your goals, or any results you've noticed

### VISUALISATION NOTES

Thoughts and reflections from this week's visualisation practices

### POSITIVE MOMENTS

Good things that you've witnessed or experienced this week

### GRATITUDE LIST

What are you thankful for this week?

Choose an exercise from the list on pages 80-81 to explore this week.
You could alternatively use this as a freewriting journal space if you prefer

**THIS WEEK'S FOCUS:**

I AM...

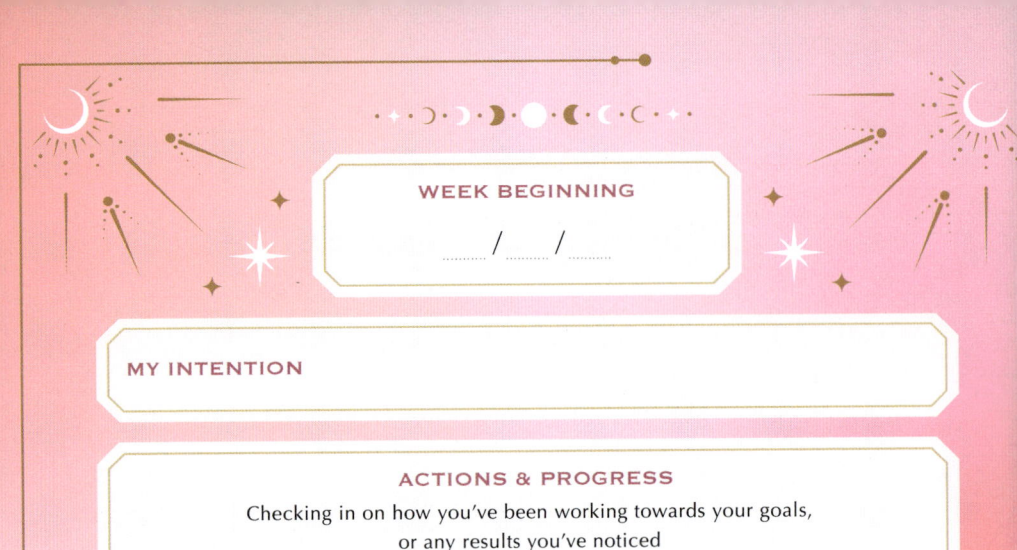

**WEEK BEGINNING**

____ / ____ / ____

**MY INTENTION**

**ACTIONS & PROGRESS**

Checking in on how you've been working towards your goals,
or any results you've noticed

**VISUALISATION NOTES**

Thoughts and reflections from this week's visualisation practices

**POSITIVE MOMENTS**

Good things that you've witnessed
or experienced this week

**GRATITUDE LIST**

What are you thankful
for this week?

Choose an exercise from the list on pages 80-81 to explore this week.
You could alternatively use this as a freewriting journal space if you prefer

**THIS WEEK'S FOCUS:**

I AM...

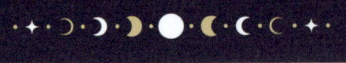

## WEEK BEGINNING
......... / ......... / .........

**MY INTENTION**

### ACTIONS & PROGRESS
Checking in on how you've been working towards your goals, or any results you've noticed

### VISUALISATION NOTES
Thoughts and reflections from this week's visualisation practices

### POSITIVE MOMENTS
Good things that you've witnessed or experienced this week

### GRATITUDE LIST
What are you thankful for this week?

Choose an exercise from the list on pages 80-81 to explore this week.
You could alternatively use this as a freewriting journal space if you prefer

**THIS WEEK'S FOCUS:**

I AM...

**WEEK BEGINNING**

......... / ......... / .........

**MY INTENTION**

**ACTIONS & PROGRESS**

Checking in on how you've been working towards your goals, or any results you've noticed

**VISUALISATION NOTES**

Thoughts and reflections from this week's visualisation practices

**POSITIVE MOMENTS**

Good things that you've witnessed or experienced this week

**GRATITUDE LIST**

What are you thankful for this week?

Choose an exercise from the list on pages 80-81 to explore this week.
You could alternatively use this as a freewriting journal space if you prefer

**THIS WEEK'S FOCUS:**

I AM...

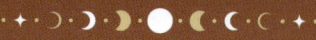

**WEEK BEGINNING**

......... / ......... / .........

## MY INTENTION

### ACTIONS & PROGRESS
Checking in on how you've been working towards your goals, or any results you've noticed

### VISUALISATION NOTES
Thoughts and reflections from this week's visualisation practices

### POSITIVE MOMENTS
Good things that you've witnessed or experienced this week

### GRATITUDE LIST
What are you thankful for this week?

Visualise your future self who has achieved your goals, and write a letter from this perspective. Envisage that version of you and describe your future life – really focusing on your feelings. Consider what advice you'd share and what support and encouragement you would offer yourself at this point in your manifestation journey

**DEAR PAST ME,**

I AM...

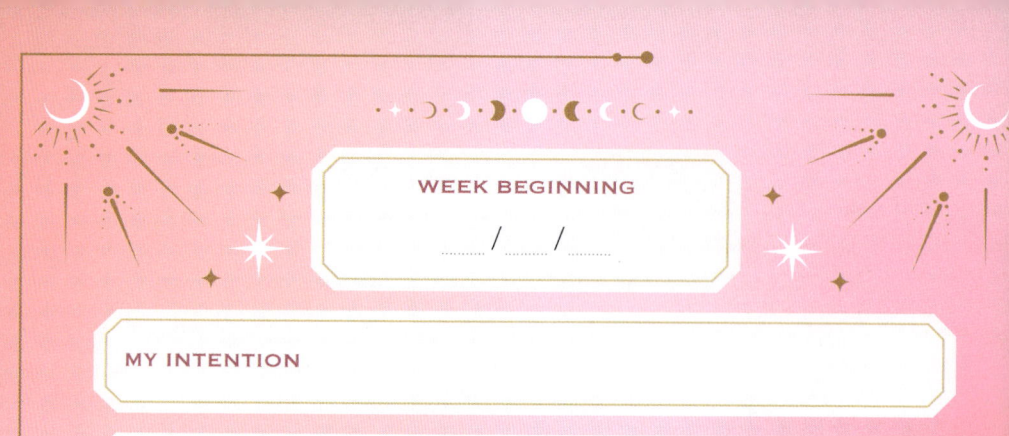

**WEEK BEGINNING**

...... / ...... / ......

**MY INTENTION**

### ACTIONS & PROGRESS
Checking in on how you've been working towards your goals, or any results you've noticed

### VISUALISATION NOTES
Thoughts and reflections from this week's visualisation practices

### POSITIVE MOMENTS
Good things that you've witnessed or experienced this week

### GRATITUDE LIST
What are you thankful for this week?

Choose an exercise from the list on pages 80-81 to explore this week.
You could alternatively use this as a freewriting journal space if you prefer

**THIS WEEK'S FOCUS:**

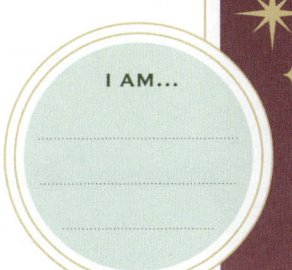

I AM...

### WEEK BEGINNING
...... / ...... / ......

## MY INTENTION

### ACTIONS & PROGRESS
Checking in on how you've been working towards your goals, or any results you've noticed

### VISUALISATION NOTES
Thoughts and reflections from this week's visualisation practices

### POSITIVE MOMENTS
Good things that you've witnessed or experienced this week

### GRATITUDE LIST
What are you thankful for this week?

Choose an exercise from the list on pages 80-81 to explore this week.
You could alternatively use this as a freewriting journal space if you prefer

**THIS WEEK'S FOCUS:**

.................................................................................................

.................................................................................................

I AM...

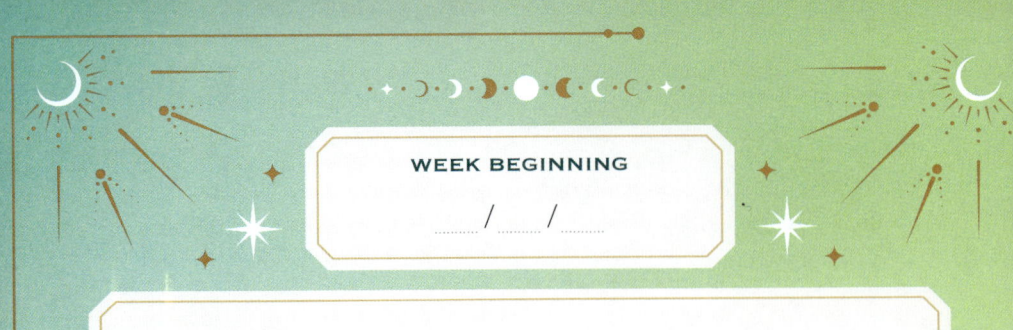

**WEEK BEGINNING**

......... / ......... / .........

**MY INTENTION**

**ACTIONS & PROGRESS**

Checking in on how you've been working towards your goals, or any results you've noticed

**VISUALISATION NOTES**

Thoughts and reflections from this week's visualisation practices

**POSITIVE MOMENTS**

Good things that you've witnessed or experienced this week

**GRATITUDE LIST**

What are you thankful for this week?

Choose an exercise from the list on pages 80-81 to explore this week.
You could alternatively use this as a freewriting journal space if you prefer

**THIS WEEK'S FOCUS:**

I AM...

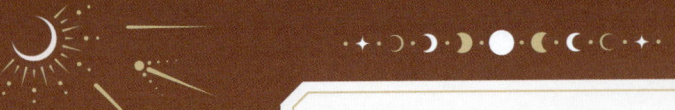

## WEEK BEGINNING
......... / ......... / .........

## MY INTENTION

### ACTIONS & PROGRESS
Checking in on how you've been working towards your goals, or any results you've noticed

### VISUALISATION NOTES
Thoughts and reflections from this week's visualisation practices

### POSITIVE MOMENTS
Good things that you've witnessed or experienced this week

### GRATITUDE LIST
What are you thankful for this week?

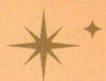

Choose an exercise from the list on pages 80-81 to explore this week.
You could alternatively use this as a freewriting journal space if you prefer

**THIS WEEK'S FOCUS:**

I AM...

**WEEK BEGINNING**

......... / ......... / .........

**MY INTENTION**

**ACTIONS & PROGRESS**

Checking in on how you've been working towards your goals, or any results you've noticed

**VISUALISATION NOTES**

Thoughts and reflections from this week's visualisation practices

**POSITIVE MOMENTS**

Good things that you've witnessed or experienced this week

**GRATITUDE LIST**

What are you thankful for this week?

Choose an exercise from the list on pages 80-81 to explore this week.
You could alternatively use this as a freewriting journal space if you prefer

**THIS WEEK'S FOCUS:**

I AM…

### WEEK BEGINNING

......... / ......... / .........

**MY INTENTION**

### ACTIONS & PROGRESS
Checking in on how you've been working towards your goals, or any results you've noticed

### VISUALISATION NOTES
Thoughts and reflections from this week's visualisation practices

### POSITIVE MOMENTS
Good things that you've witnessed or experienced this week

### GRATITUDE LIST
What are you thankful for this week?

Choose an exercise from the list on pages 80-81 to explore this week.
You could alternatively use this as a freewriting journal space if you prefer

**THIS WEEK'S FOCUS:**

I AM...

### WEEK BEGINNING
...... / ...... / ......

## MY INTENTION

### ACTIONS & PROGRESS
Checking in on how you've been working towards your goals, or any results you've noticed

### VISUALISATION NOTES
Thoughts and reflections from this week's visualisation practices

### POSITIVE MOMENTS
Good things that you've witnessed or experienced this week

### GRATITUDE LIST
What are you thankful for this week?

Choose an exercise from the list on pages 80-81 to explore this week.
You could alternatively use this as a freewriting journal space if you prefer

**THIS WEEK'S FOCUS:**

I AM…

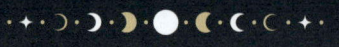

## WEEK BEGINNING

........... / ........... / ...........

**MY INTENTION**

### ACTIONS & PROGRESS

Checking in on how you've been working towards your goals, or any results you've noticed

### VISUALISATION NOTES

Thoughts and reflections from this week's visualisation practices

### POSITIVE MOMENTS

Good things that you've witnessed or experienced this week

### GRATITUDE LIST

What are you thankful for this week?

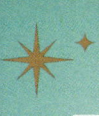

Choose an exercise from the list on pages 80-81 to explore this week.
You could alternatively use this as a freewriting journal space if you prefer

**THIS WEEK'S FOCUS:**

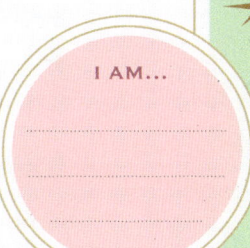

I AM…

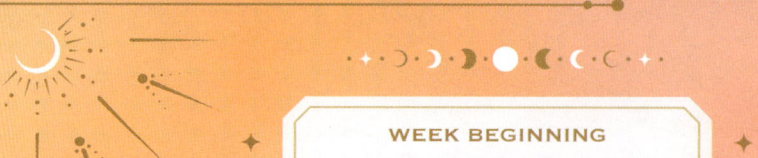

## WEEK BEGINNING
...... / ...... / ......

## MY INTENTION

### ACTIONS & PROGRESS
Checking in on how you've been working towards your goals, or any results you've noticed

### VISUALISATION NOTES
Thoughts and reflections from this week's visualisation practices

### POSITIVE MOMENTS
Good things that you've witnessed or experienced this week

### GRATITUDE LIST
What are you thankful for this week?

Choose an exercise from the list on pages 80-81 to explore this week.
You could alternatively use this as a freewriting journal space if you prefer

**THIS WEEK'S FOCUS:**

I AM...

**WEEK BEGINNING**

......... / ......... / .........

**MY INTENTION**

### ACTIONS & PROGRESS

Checking in on how you've been working towards your goals, or any results you've noticed

### VISUALISATION NOTES

Thoughts and reflections from this week's visualisation practices

### POSITIVE MOMENTS

Good things that you've witnessed or experienced this week

### GRATITUDE LIST

What are you thankful for this week?

Choose an exercise from the list on pages 80-81 to explore this week.
You could alternatively use this as a freewriting journal space if you prefer

**THIS WEEK'S FOCUS:**

## WEEK BEGINNING

..... / ..... / .....

## MY INTENTION

### ACTIONS & PROGRESS

Checking in on how you've been working towards your goals, or any results you've noticed

### VISUALISATION NOTES

Thoughts and reflections from this week's visualisation practices

### POSITIVE MOMENTS

Good things that you've witnessed or experienced this week

### GRATITUDE LIST

What are you thankful for this week?

Choose an exercise from the list on pages 80-81 to explore this week.
You could alternatively use this as a freewriting journal space if you prefer

**THIS WEEK'S FOCUS:**

I AM...

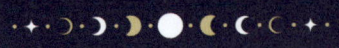

### WEEK BEGINNING
...... / ...... / ......

## MY INTENTION

### ACTIONS & PROGRESS
Checking in on how you've been working towards your goals, or any results you've noticed

### VISUALISATION NOTES
Thoughts and reflections from this week's visualisation practices

### POSITIVE MOMENTS
Good things that you've witnessed or experienced this week

### GRATITUDE LIST
What are you thankful for this week?

Choose an exercise from the list on pages 80-81 to explore this week.
You could alternatively use this as a freewriting journal space if you prefer

**THIS WEEK'S FOCUS:**

I AM...

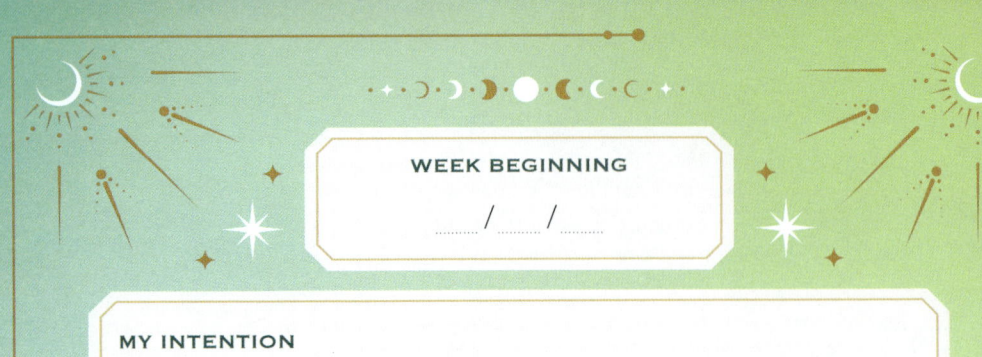

### WEEK BEGINNING

...... / ...... / ......

**MY INTENTION**

### ACTIONS & PROGRESS

Checking in on how you've been working towards your goals, or any results you've noticed

### VISUALISATION NOTES

Thoughts and reflections from this week's visualisation practices

### POSITIVE MOMENTS

Good things that you've witnessed or experienced this week

### GRATITUDE LIST

What are you thankful for this week?

Visualise your future self who has achieved your goals, and write a letter from this perspective. Envisage that version of you and describe your future life – really focusing on your feelings. Consider what advice you'd share and what support and encouragement you would offer yourself at this point in your manifestation journey

**DEAR PAST ME,**

I AM…

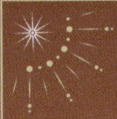

# End-of-year reflections

**LOOK BACK OVER THE LAST 52 WEEKS AND APPRECIATE HOW FAR YOU'VE COME**

WORDS | JULIE BASSETT

As we come to the end of a full year of writing in this journal, it's time to take a moment to reflect on what you've achieved.

If you started out new to manifestation, think about what has changed since you introduced it into your life. What have you learned about yourself? Has manifestation become part of your daily routine? Maybe you already had some experience with manifestation before now, so you might want to think about whether you've managed to deepen your practice or make big moves towards your goals. No matter where you are on your manifestation pathway, you should be proud of yourself for being consistent and taking time to fill out your journal and map your intentions.

Think about how far you've come. Success isn't always based on whether you've managed to manifest the goals you set at the start. Any progress you've made deserves to be celebrated – every step is a step closer. It might be that you've noticed other positive changes that you weren't expecting. Manifestation might have given you a clearer focus, a happier outlook, a more positive mindset or greater self-esteem, and these are all incredible aspects of the journey you should recognise and give yourself credit for.

While you reflect, think about what you're grateful for. You may feel gratitude towards the practices that have become part of your life; towards yourself for putting your intentions into action; towards the people who have supported you along the way; or towards the opportunities you've taken.

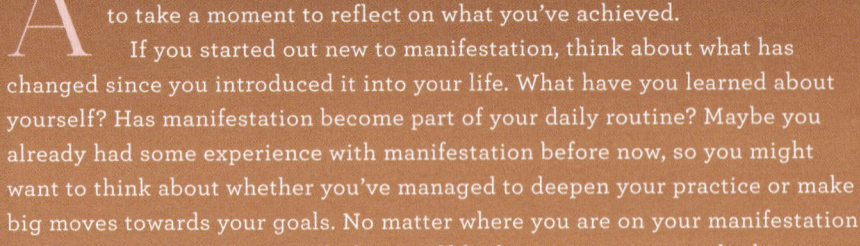

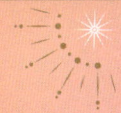

# YOUR SUCCESSES

Look back through your journal entries and identify your top five successes for the year. If you've achieved one of your big goals, this is definitely something to highlight. But don't forget about the small wins along the way too; these are just as important to acknowledge. Think about the key steps and actions you took that helped you achieve each success.

**SUCCESS 1**
**KEY STEPS**




**SUCCESS 2**
**KEY STEPS**




**SUCCESS 3**
**KEY STEPS**




**SUCCESS 4**
**KEY STEPS**




**SUCCESS 5**
**KEY STEPS**

# CHALLENGES & LESSONS

Nothing goes to plan all the time. Throughout this year, you're sure to have had challenges, setbacks and obstacles. Think about some of the challenges you've faced, how you overcame them and what lessons you've learned for the future.

**CHALLENGE 1**
**HOW I OVERCAME IT**


**LESSON(S) LEARNED**


**CHALLENGE 2**
**HOW I OVERCAME IT**


**LESSON(S) LEARNED**


**CHALLENGE 3**
**HOW I OVERCAME IT**


**LESSON(S) LEARNED**

# PATTERNS

Have you noticed any patterns that have influenced your manifestation practice, whether positively or negatively? For example: starting a new habit has made you more positive; skipping your affirmations has led to negative self-talk; daily journalling has improved your self-confidence. Use this blank space to write down anything that comes to mind and join connected points with arrows so you can see the patterns emerge.

**COMPARE PAST & PRESENT**
Spend some time revisiting your 'Dear past me…' letters (pages 107, 133, 159 and 185). Perhaps you feel a little closer to your imagined 'future self' now, channelling that positive energy back to your past self.

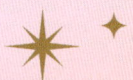

# AREAS FOR IMPROVEMENT

Write about what you could do differently next year to make your manifestation practice more successful. For example, do you need to be more consistent? Are there any mental blocks or obstacles affecting your practice? Do you need to introduce a different manifestation technique? Be honest, as it can help you move forward into the next 12 months.

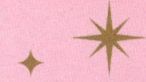

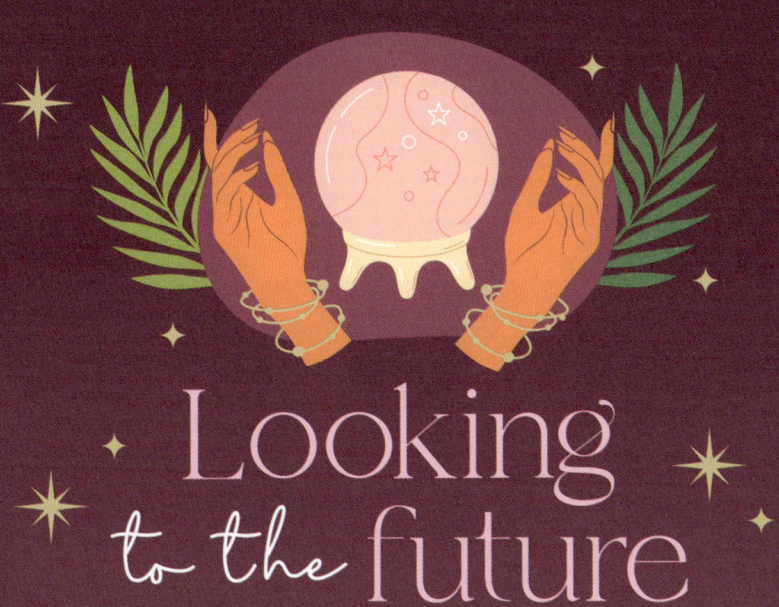

# Looking to the future

Your journey doesn't end here. You can take all your learnings and reflections from the past year, and feed them into the next 52 weeks. Manifestation can be a lifelong pursuit, helping you to keep working towards the life you want for yourself.

It might be that you go into a new year with the same goals and intentions. Think about how far you've moved towards those goals already and how much you have achieved. Then you can consider what you still have left to do, and update your intentions and actions to keep moving forwards. You may have learned that there are certain obstacles that will always be there, which helps you to shift your actions to make way for them.

Alternatively, you may be looking to introduce a new set of intentions, whether that's because you've already met your initial goals, or because your priorities have changed and you want to move in a different direction. This is the perfect time to realign your manifestation practice if you want to. This can be a fresh start if that's what you need.

Either way, it's a good idea to think about a new mantra or affirmation that sums up what you hope for in the next 12 months. This can act as a singular focus point that combines all your intentions into one overarching theme. Take this opportunity to set your intentions for the next year on the following page, and start to manifest and shape your future just the way you want it.

# Next year

TAKE SOME TIME TO CONSIDER YOUR GOALS AND INTENTIONS FOR THE YEAR AHEAD, AND WHAT STEPS YOU CAN TAKE TOWARDS MAKING THEM A REALITY

Congratulations on completing your journal! We hope you continue to employ the techniques you've learned here to keep manifesting the life you want.

# Manifesting Journal

**Future PLC** Quay House, The Ambury, Bath, BA1 1UA

### Editorial
Editor **Jacqueline Snowden**
Art Editor **Katy Stokes**
Head of Art & Design **Greg Whitaker**
Editorial Director **Jon White**
Managing Director **Grainne McKenna**

### Contributors
Sarah Bankes, Julie Bassett, Josephine Hall, Harriet Knight, Beate Triantafilidis

### Cover images
Getty Images

### Advertising
Media packs are available on request
Commercial Director **Clare Dove**

### International
Head of Print Licensing **Rachel Shaw**
licensing@futurenet.com
www.futurecontenthub.com

### Circulation
Head of Newstrade **Tim Mathers**

### Production
Head of Production **Mark Constance**
Production Project Manager **Matthew Eglinton**
Advertising Production Manager **Joanne Crosby**
Digital Editions Controller **Jason Hudson**
Production Managers **Keely Miller, Nola Cokely, Vivienne Calvert, Fran Twentyman**

Printed in the UK

**Distributed by** Marketforce – www.marketforce.co.uk
For enquiries, please email: mfcommunications@futurenet.com

**GPSR EU RP (for authorities only)**
eucomply OÜ Pärnu mnt 139b-14 11317, Tallinn, Estonia
hello@eucompliancepartner.com, +3375690241

**The Manifesting Journal First Edition (LBZ7030)**
© 2025 Future Publishing Limited

We are committed to only using magazine paper which is derived from responsibly managed, certified forestry and chlorine-free manufacture. The paper in this bookazine was sourced and produced from sustainable managed forests, conforming to strict environmental and socioeconomic standards.

All contents © 2025 Future Publishing Limited or published under licence. All rights reserved. No part of this magazine may be used, stored, transmitted or reproduced in any way without the prior written permission of the publisher. Future Publishing Limited (company number 2008885) is registered in England and Wales. Registered office: Quay House, The Ambury, Bath BA1 1UA. All information contained in this publication is for information only and is, as far as we are aware, correct at the time of going to press. Future cannot accept any responsibility for errors or inaccuracies in such information. You are advised to contact manufacturers and retailers directly with regard to the price of products/services referred to in this publication. Apps and websites mentioned in this publication are not under our control. We are not responsible for their contents or any other changes or updates to them. This magazine is fully independent and not affiliated in any way with the companies mentioned herein.

# FUTURE
Connectors.
Creators.
Experience Makers.

Future plc is a public company quoted on the London Stock Exchange (symbol: FUTR)
www.futureplc.com

Chief Executive Officer **Kevin Li Ying**
Non-Executive Chairman **Richard Huntingford**
Chief Financial Officer **Sharjeel Suleman**

Tel +44 (0)1225 442 244